Full of Sound and Fury

Suffering With Misophonia

Shaylynn Hayes

FULL OF SOUND AND FURY: SUFFERING WITH MISOPHONIA
SECOND EDITION © 2016
was written by Shaylynn Hayes and is intended to help sufferers and their loved ones come to terms with Misophonia. This books intent is to get as much information out there as possible and to raise awareness in doing so.

While copyright dictates that no part of this book can be re-printed or re- produced in any form without permission, sharing the information is encouraged. You may use up to 500 words (about 2 pages) as a brief excerpt for blog posts or other mediums of sharing information, providing proper authorship is noted. If you would like to reprint larger sections, please contact the author. If you would like to share the information presented in this book please use proper citation.

You may share your purchased copy with your friends. In-fact, I encourage that you do so. Awareness is the main purpose of this book, and I would like the information to be accessible. However, if the person likes the book, I would love if they purchased a copy, or supported our Facebook page.

Distributed directly through www.Misophoniainternational.com.

Copies of this book may be found through major providers through an ebook form.

Editing and Proofreading by Victoria MacNeil-LeBlanc and Danielle Waterman

Design, cover, and formatting by Shaylynn Hayes
Foreword by Jennifer Jo-Brout

ISBN-13: 978-1517018702
ISBN-10: 1517018706

Life's but a walking shadow, a poor player
That struts and frets his hour upon the stage
And then is heard no more.
It is a tale
Told by an idiot, full of sound and fury,
Signifying nothing.

- Shakespeare

Dedication

Many suffer in silence, every day.
This book is for those that need
to know that they're not alone.
And, to Jennifer, because she
"gets it".

Welcome to the Revised and Updated 2nd Edition

When I first set out to write *Full of Sound and Fury*, I never knew where my life was going to take me. I can't believe it's only been a year. In that year, I have embarked on a challenging, yet fulfilling journey. I have discovered what it means, to me, to suffer with a lesser-known disorder, and I have realized that true empowerment is not only personal, but comes from a place of "suffering" or at least trial and tribulation.

The past year has been one of change - growth - and of course, hard work. As I said, when I started this book, I had no idea what it was going to mean to me. It was a way to experience my disorder, and to help others share their stories. Today, it is much much more.

It may seem soon to write a new edition - after all, the book is merely a year old, from its start. But, you see, the world of research and of disorders is ever-moving - it is a fluid process that runs freely and it crashes like waves, all around us. I am nowhere near the same person that wrote this book - and as such, I need to ensure that it reflects my most current views. This may not be entirely possible, since things change so fast, but I assure you, I am trying.

How could I have known when I asked Jennifer to read my book that she would become one of the most influential people in my life? How could I have known that the secret to getting research done was to work for it? Yes, we have a long way to go, but the groundwork has been laid. Sufferers, like you, like me, we're not only the reason for suffering, we're the ones who need to take action.

I used to be in the dark. I was alone, and I was scared. After-all, no one seemed to know what was wrong with me. My mother was at her wits end - our relationship on the fritz. My friendships were tested. Who wants to hang out with the "crabby girl"?

The reasons for these changes alone should help convince you that Misophonia research is possible, and probable. I'll tell you why and how you can help later, in a newly added chapter, but for now, I'll just inform you of all the things that have changed. It's actually really exciting, and I can't believe I'm a part of it.

Whether or not Misophonia is actually a sub-set of SPD (such as SOR, or sensory over-regulation) remains to be seen. Misophonia, SPD, and other sensory related issues can seem as though they have stolen your life. Mental disorders such as OCD, Depression, Anxiety, ADHD, or others can hijack the situation and turn it into a bitter pill to swallow. But, it's not entirely hopeless. Actually, I'd be willing to say it's not hopeless at all.

When I first discovered that I had Misophonia I spent a lot of time in my house. I became isolated by my strong desire to protect myself. After all, who wouldn't want to avoid a traumatic situation? Though, as this behaviour continued I noticed a pattern. The more I tried to avoid triggers, the more I was triggered. Not only that, the severity was growing. At first, I attributed this to a hopeless reality: this disorder was getting worse and would eventually take over all aspects of my life.

In the past month I have done several things that I never expected to do again. Trapped and isolated in my disorder, I had waged war against all unnecessary public behavior. I mean, I shopped, but that's not exactly a sincere socialization process. I have gone to a restaurant 6 or 7 times, previously I avoided this like the plague – now, I'm less inclined to say no to a friend. After all, life's short. I went to the movies. A 3D movie with popcorn eaters and all (luckily chewing is a rare trigger for me, but still, I got past the anxiety).

There is not going to be a 'one size fits all' cure for Misophonia. The disorder, like SPD, is complex. Each and every sufferer is going to have their own past experiences, their own desires, and their own fears. Work with that. Identify who you are and where you're triggered. Do you feel worse when you're tired/dehydrated? Are certain foods making it worse? Explore and listen to your body – literally. It may be trying to have a conversation with you.

Misophonia can seem strange to people who have never heard of it. I know that before I knew the name, I merely thought I was "going crazy". Of course, I now know that there has been research on similar conditions for the past 30 years.

The name may be new, but the disorder itself is not as rare and unthinkable as I first believed.

One year ago, I decided that it was time to write a book that highlighted the feeling of Misophonia sufferers. What I didn't know - it was going to connect me to the entire Research situation, and that I'd eventually have to shake off my biases and dedicate myself to being an advocate. In the first edition I swear that I am "not" an advocate. But, I've learned to embrace the title. We need to advocate for ourselves and for each other.

Foreword

Shaylynn Hayes has written a candid and informative book about Misophonia. When I first began to chat with Shaylynn, she reminded me very much of one of my daughters, who is the same age. I am very moved by Ms. Hayes' ability to write about this disorder, as she shares her own experiences and also takes great care to be objective in presenting both a variety of case studies and different viewpoints about the nature of Misophonia.

Ms. Hayes takes Misophonia awareness very seriously and has dedicated her time, talent and resources to her book. For Ms. Hayes, Misophonia symptoms began at age 16 and as she got older, worsened. For my daughter they began as far back as I remember.

Over 15 years ago a most amazing 5 year old child looked at me and asked "Mommy, can you fix my brain?". She asked me this because she was overly sensitive to noises. These sounds were not necessarily loud, they were not necessarily high-pitched, and they were not necessarily noises that other people found aversive or frightening. Yet, for my daughter these noises were horrifying. They were frightening. They made her angry. My sweet daughter, who was highly social, who loved people, enjoyed being around others and was highly empathic was stopped dead in her tracks by certain sounds. She became overwhelmed, she had to leave the room, she screamed, she cried, and often I would find her weeping with her hands over her ears in her closet hiding. Could I fix her brain? I couldn't even figure out what sounds were bothering her, never mind why or how to fix the problem.

This began a long journey that has in essence for me, begun again. When my daughter was 5, after taking her for treatment to a bevy of psychiatrists who misdiagnosed, and mistreated her, I finally figured out what was going on. I was lucky (or perhaps unlucky). I suffer from the same condition. Yet, I don't have it as badly, or at least I didn't when I was younger. Like many others, my symptoms have worsened over time. Yet, having the same symptoms allowed me to figure out what was going on with my daughter.

At the time, around 1996, I was in graduate school studying to be a psychologist, and yet nobody could help my daughter with this "new condition" which was then called Sensory Processing Disorder (SPD). One subtype of the disorder, Sensory Over Responsivity (SOR) describes children who misinterpret sensory information, and react to it as thought it were aversive. This condition, which includes extreme aversive reactivity to sensory stimuli including sounds, was being studied under the name SPD by Occupational Therapists, not by psychologists and not by psychiatrists. Ground breaking research by Dr. Lucy Miller and colleagues revealed that auditory and other sensory stimuli is misinterpreted by the brain and causes the sufferer to go into fight/flight. In addition, once the fight/flight response is activated, the part of the nervous system that should put "the brakes on fight/flight", is less efficient. That is, children who are overly sensitive to sensory stimuli react more severely to noise (and other sensory information) and are deficient in calming down.

Fast forward, approximately 18 years later and I have the pleasure of getting to know Ms. Hayes through Facebook groups dedicated to Misophonia. Ms. Hayes is a young lady seemingly mature beyond her years, struggling to advocate for and understand this condition. Certain noises and visual triggers make her feel overloaded, out of control, enraged, physically ill, frightened, and altogether dysregulated. She, like my daughter, like me, and like so many others who have now formed groups on social media, are demanding answers.

Shaylynn, is a young lady who has taken advocacy into her own hands by writing a book, a commendable action!

SPD Sensory Over Responsivity? Misophonia or Selective Sound Sensitivity Syndrome? This is not my first "rodeo" with this same or related disorder(s) in which certain sounds (soft ones, repetitive ones, loud ones, ones that go unnoticed by others) are the bane of peoples' existence. I've seen "up close" how the DSM-V rejects SPD and other important disorders for reasons that seem absurd. I've seen first hand how research does and doesn't get done. I've seen how research is, or is not translated into effective therapy.

For me, this is "take two" with what I always called "auditory over- responsivity" but which is now called Misophonia.

I hope that Ms. Hayes will be an inspiration to others that we must take matters into our own hands. We must not wait for "them to do research" or wait until "they find a cure". There is no "they". We are the "they".

Ms. Hayes, with her high intelligence and ability to reason, fairly and objectively wrote a book that presents differing points of view, while simultaneously revealing real and painful stories of sufferers, including her own.

I hope that people will follow Shaylynn's example and advocate, raise awareness, write books, and comment every time you see an article written about Misophonia that you don't agree with.

Jennifer Jo Brout -PsyD

What Is Misophonia?

Misophonia, pronunciation debated, is known to be a neurological disorder. The term Misophonia, literally translating to "hatred of sound", refers to a negative reaction caused by sounds that immediately and involuntarily enrage the sufferer. While the name reflects only sounds, many sufferers are triggered by visuals as well. The condition often leads to isolation, depressed feelings, heightened anxiety, complicated work life and school life, and even family and relationship problems. If you are triggered by the mention of trigger sources, please feel free to bypass the following mention of triggers. Most triggers are repetitive actions, and several visual triggers are related to audial triggers. It's important to note that depending on the person, there can be hundreds of individual triggers. The below are merely examples of common triggers.

Audial Trigger Examples
- Whistling
- Snoring
- Pen-tapping
- Foot-tapping
- Chewing
- Heavy Breathing

Visual Trigger Examples
- Leg shaking

- Swaying
- Bouncing
- Chewing
- Hand movements
- Foot movements
- Pen clicking

A research study of Misophonia interviewed sufferers. According to the researchers, those with Misophonia, "reported feeling offended or violated by these sounds to the point where negative thoughts such as 'I hate this person,' 'Stop it, I can't stand it,' and 'Don't you know what you sound like?' enter their minds" (Edelstein). This reaction is typical for Misophonia. Having felt it myself, I can say that no words can describe the intense emotions that happens if you are at the far end of the spectrum.

According to the study "Misophonia: physiological investigations and case descriptions", Misophonia is: "a relatively unexplored chronic condition in which a person experiences autonomic arousal (analogous to an involuntary "fight-or-flight" response) to certain innocuous or repetitive sounds such as chewing, pen clicking, and lip smacking. Misophonics report anxiety, panic, and rage when exposed to trigger sounds, compromising their ability to complete everyday tasks and engage in healthy and normal social interaction" (Edelstein)

While this summary leaves out the visual triggers, it is

an adequate description of the disorder. Misophonia can be so intense that it interrupts daily life, and has caused some sufferers to fall into a deep depression. Sufferers have also expressed reactions from certain fabrics or the sensation of touching certain objects. Other sensory involved reactions have been documented in cases, and it is clear that these are related. Thus, the name "Misophonia" has gotten some flack from both sufferers and members of the medical community. The name "Misophonia," meaning hatred of sound, may seem fine to people who identify the disorder with hearing and audial triggers. However, many of the sufferers have problems with visuals, as well as tactile problems.

Though some doctors have come up with medical terms and definitions for the disorder there is no solid evidence or facts that give a solid explanation of what Misophonia is.

What we do know is that it should not be assumed that those with Misophonia should force exposure to their triggers in order to "get used to them." Any current evidence points to exposure causing the condition to worsen over time. It is important that people with Misophonia realize that they should not feel guilty for having the disorder, should know when enough is enough, and to leave the situation if they feel that it's necessary. Of course, many triggers cannot be avoided entirely, but it is okay to avoid situations that may expose one's self to a high number of them. It is of no use to continue exposing yourself to triggers repeatedly, especially if the reward of the situation or activity is quite low.

Misophonia can feel like a trap. We have been thrown against our will, and without any warrant, in a suffocating prison. Some have suffered their entire lives, and the more fortunate, for a few years. Regardless, the condition is the same. It is important to note that there are several degrees of Misophonia.

A lot of the time, a person that has Misophonia ends up isolating his or her self from the rest of the world. It can be a heavy burden to be triggered by numerous people and normal activities. This leads to sadness, anxiety, and a lowered quality of life. This is especially prominent in individuals who have other disorders – especially mood disorders. Misophonia can cause grief.

Misophonia can do a lot of damage on personal relationships. Misophonia has an impact not only on the sufferer; it also affects the friends, family, and romantic partners of the individual. It can cause a lot of arguments and fights, and is especially difficult when there is a lack of understanding between persons.

My Story

When I first discovered what "Misophonia" is I had an entirely different story to tell. I was relieved there was a name. I was also scared that I have a disorder that seems to be under-researched, and would be at risk to be stigmatized.

Most people that I have talked to with Misophonia have been suffering since they were children. However, I am one of the late-bloomers. Regardless of when it came to be, Misophonia is an extremely isolating disorder. I was 16 when I showed my first symptoms, but they were not strong. It wasn't until 19 when the full force of Misophonia hit me like a freight train. Since then, I have felt its wrath clasp around my throat, taking over several aspects of my life. My first blog post on Misophonia was written before I even knew there was a name – before I had anything to go on. I remember writing in frustration, tears not far off, as I wondered why I was so messed up. Why, all of a sudden, I was having so much trouble with sights and sounds. When I first came across Misophonia, I described it as ruining my life. I didn't understand why, but these everyday movements and sounds were turning normal situations into a terrible prison.

I attributed my first triggers to an anxiety disorder, as well as major depressive disorder. Small movements, or rock-ing back and forth was enough to cause near panic attacks. If a desk was not sitting on the floor properly, I would lose it. If a classmate was making loud, distracting noises, I'd complain to the teacher. It didn't always get me far, but if they didn't help, I'd leave. I wasn't the most attentive student in high school.

On January 27th, 2014, I wrote a post expressing my confusion and rage, in regards to what I now know as Misophonia. Please bare in mind that this was written before I had any idea what Misophonia was. The title was "I don't know what to do". Below, it is recopied in full.

When I first came to university I didn't remember why I had been so distracted and annoyed in high school. Homework isn't hard, the reading is fine. What I can't deal with is the burden that my anxiety can be in a classroom environment. Half of the time I have a scowl on my face in class and probably come off as a bit of a condescending witch. Whenever people whistle, click their pen, or shake their legs, it's extremely distracting for me and for a reason I cannot explain it sends me into a horrible state. Leg twitching in my peripheral vision has literally brought me to tears. I'm so frustrated that I can't just "get over it". I understand restless leg syndrome is a real thing but so is the anxiety that I suffer every time I enter a classroom. I understand that it would be rude to approach somebody and ask them to please stop torturing me.

Instead, I often stew and try not to get upset but instead I usually just end up irrationally angry. Often times I can actually feel the vibrations on the floor from people shaking behind me, even if they're far away. A couple of weeks ago I started hyperventilating when somebody was whistling. Why? The sharp noise was so unbearable to me. I honestly don't know what I'm supposed to do about this. Breathing exercises, telling myself it's out of my control and "thinking positive" are hopeless.

I don't want to constantly glare at my friends like they're the worst thing in the world just because they're shaking their feet. I'm actually sorry it bugs me this much but I can't stop. Sometimes I find myself sitting in my room anxious about going to class just because of my triggers. I just feel alone in this and that I must sound ridiculous to others. Aside from hiding in my room wearing ear plugs and only ever communicating via skype I'm not sure of a fix to this.

My first "real" trigger was whistling. I would go into a rage and nearly cry whenever faced with it. Some people would whistle on purpose, because they did not understand the severity of my reaction. I remember being upset for hours after this would happen, and that confused me a lot. Then, one day my mother's foot shaking really started to bother me. Soon after, the sound of singing and country music really sent me over the edge. This caused a lot of fights and confusion – why was I so intolerant? It made no sense.

On March 14th, 2015, I described my feelings in a blog post entitled "The Agony of Misophonia".

"Everybody gets annoyed by certain noises."

"You just need to get over it, you can't change the way the world works."

Welcome to Misophonia. Like other conditions, those of us who suffer get to live day to day with the horror of explaining it to others. We're those "crazy" people who give you an angry glare when you click your pen, chew too loudly, or shake your foot. Some are perpetually angry,nitpick and we are hard to be around sometimes. We don't want to be that way. Believe me, I haven't chosen this neurological hell. I want to sit in my own apartment and not cry day and night because the guy upstairs is walking too loud. I want to go on a bus and not have to worry about the guy whistling. I want to live my life.

It is possible though, to live a fulfilling life with Misophonia. If you're able to see it for what it is and be proactive - you can manage your mood, and ensure that even when you are triggered, it doesn't cause a catastrophic event.

A large problem with Misophonia is the lack of public awareness. I've been advocating to fix that in every way I can. There's not a lot I can do – but I can share my personal experiences. From what I gather about Misophonia – there's a lot of instances that are the same for a lot of us. However, it's important to note that everybody is triggered by an array of different things. If one person with Misophonia hates whistling – the next might be affected more by chomping or chewing. Breathing, itself, can even be seriously bothersome to sufferers.

I must note that I also have ADHD, Major Depressive Disorder and Generalized Anxiety Disorder. These conditions can seriously impact my personal reactions. However, they may merely be part of a bigger picture - do we have several conditions - or is misdiagnosis so widespread that labels are overcoming factual analysis of the brain and the human condition.

We're not all the same, so that makes it even harder to

raise awareness. However, regardless of what a person is triggered by, we're still triggered, and it's bad.

It's hard for me not to think of Shakespeare's quote "full of sound and fury signifying nothing". This quote perfectly expresses the disorder, and that's why it's been incorporated into the title. There's no logical reason to freak out – we can feel crazy, guilty, and downright ridiculous. It's full of fury. We're angry, we're furious – we're in a whirlwind of emotion that usually takes a turn toward self-inflicted misery, or worse, anger directed at the sound. The simple clicking of a pen can feel like we're trapped in a cavern with a jackhammer.

What happens when I'm triggered: The sound comes at me like a crashing wave. Before the trigger I'm usually fine. I'm sitting or standing there living my life, minding my own business and then – whoosh – Tsunami. I can't breathe; I'm angry – terrified, pissed off. I want the offender to stop. I blame them for all my problems. Words like "rude", "annoying", and "horrible" describe that person. I try to isolate myself. If it's a visual trigger (like leg shaking) I try to hide it from my vision. If it's audial, I put in earplugs. But I know it's there. I can feel its presence in the room. I shake from within. The anxiety builds and I want to throw up – and at that point all I can do is run away. Sometimes I shake violently and I cry. Sometimes I sleep for hours when I should be in school. I feel self-pity. I want to live my life. Then, I feel anger, depression, anxiety. Why does this disorder exist? Why me?

On the "support" forums I have seen people try to describe Misophonia as a "rage" disorder. I have heard people say we are "violent". I do not believe that to be true. Regardless of my triggers and their extremities, I have never once wanted to hurt somebody for triggering me. Perhaps I see them as a threat and feel deeply insulted, but I do not contemplate violence. If a person has "Misophonia" and is accompanied by this extreme rage and has contemplated hurting another, they should immediately seek out medical help. This is probably an anger issue that stems from other parts of your life and should be addressed.

Misophonics, for lack of a better term, are not just angry or irritated. We cannot handle things because our brain is unable to filter information - therefore we are assaulted by our own sensory systems.

I wish I could tell you that there's a cure. I want to tell you that it gets easier, and that it's all just some silly misunderstanding. I can't do that. That's why I'm pushing for advocacy. The world needs to know that we're not getting angry on purpose. It's not something to make fun of or use against a person. It's real, it's terrible, and it's ruining our lives.

Interviews With Sufferers

People whose lives are affected by Misophonia filled out the following interviews graciously. All of the answers are unaltered, with the exception of spelling or grammar, and are 100% honest. The opinions within these interviews are that of the interviewee. The question form was the same for each individual. The following interviews are not presented in any given order. I am so thankful to the people who chose to share their experiences with Misophonia in this book.

Name: Adam Johnson

Age: 40

Sex: M

Country: USA

State/Province/Territory: Michigan

At what age did you start to have triggers for Misophonia?

I have a clear memory at about 7 years old with a single trigger.

What are your top 5 triggers?

Chewing of any kind (both auditory and visual)

Breathing

Fingers on keyboards

Sipping / slurping (assuming this is different than chewing, and auditory only)

Bright lights (reflections, point sources, etc.)

What is worse, visual triggers or audial triggers?

Audial is much more severe. Bright lights are right behind and are a migraine trigger as well.

When did you learn that there was a name for your condition and other sufferers?

About 2 years ago I found the term Selective Sound Sensitivity Syndrome online. This led me to Misophonia.

How did it feel to learn that there were other people like

you?

It made me feel better for sure. This sensitivity can make me hard to live and work with sometimes, so it made me feel less... crazy?

How do you cope with this disorder?

When eating with family and friends, I make sure to have music playing to minimize the eating sounds. Restaurants are chosen for the same reason. I wear headphones a lot. A whole lot. This drowns out keyboards in offices, people on airplanes, etc. For the light sensitivity part, I wear sunglasses a lot, keep offices and living spaces free of bright lights, and arrange computer screens to not reflect.

Are your family and friends supportive?

No. It's not an easy thing to grasp, and I just seem like I'm being annoyed.

Are you afraid to confront a person when they are triggering you?

Unfortunately, I confront often. I ask people (and many times strangers) to stop slurping coffee, to chew with their mouths closed, to spit out their gum, etc.

If a person does not respect your condition, how do you react?

I have to leave before I take their coffee, food, gum away.

Do you have other disorders that worsen your Misophonia?

When I'm feeling "migraine-prone" which I consider unusually light- sensitive and not far from triggering a migraine, my sensitivity to all things intensifies.

Do you think the name suits the disorder? Why? Why not?

Yes. Sound is often my enemy and I therefore hate it. This is unfortunate for the people creating the sounds...

Are you on any drugs that do or do not help (antidepressants, anti- psychotics, etc.)?

None.

What do you think could be done to raise awareness?

Perhaps some legitimate interviews on mainstream media, with legitimate medical professionals.

Explain the reaction when faced with a trigger:

I first try to just ignore it, to focus on something else. If it continues and I start to feel either pain and/or anger, I see if it's something I can fix delicately, or if I need to take myself out of the situation. If I'm 'stuck' in the environment and glaring at someone isn't working, and I can't discretely plug my ears a last resort is to try to explain that sounds are hurting me. Either way, the longer the sound goes on, the more I go from mildly annoyed and patient, to pained, to downright angry and irrational.

Name: Simone Zoffmann Johansen

Age: 18

Sex: Female

Country: Denmark

State/Province/Territory: Vordingborg

At what age did you start to have triggers for Misophonia?

I first really noticed when I was 14 years old, which is 4 years ago.

What are your top 5 triggers?

It's hard for me to categorize the triggers in numbers, but my worst triggers are:

People chewing – basically everything is annoying me about that.

People making a noise with candy bags, chips bags, etc.

People using their mouse pad on their computers or using their keyboard People playing with a pen, clicking it etc.

People making a noise with their fingers on a table rhythmically.

What is worse, visual triggers or audial triggers?

Audial triggers are for sure the worst kinds of triggers, but the hard thing is that, when you start getting anxiety of audial triggers, visual triggers can be just as horrible as audial triggers, because inside your head – you can hear the audial triggers when you get visually triggered.

When did you learn that there was a name for your condition and other sufferers?

About a half year ago, by a coincidence, I found a Danish name for the condition, which is called "to be particularly sensitive." It was at first a huge relief. I read a whole lot about it and it was fantastic to find out that I wasn't the only one who was triggered by something. Someday, again by a coincidence, one of my classmates (who I have yelled at many times, because he has triggered me with his noises) came and showed me a so- called meme, from Facebook which said "getting angry at people when hear them breathing or eating is called 'Misophonia', which is an actual brain disorder." Then I researched a lot about Misophonia and found out that this was the word, which described everything that I felt inside.

How did it feel to learn that there were other people like you?

It was a huge relief. Day in and day out for at least 4 years, I have been called a lot of things for being so rude, angry, parochial and hysterical. Suddenly there was an explanation, which I, more than anyone else, had been searching for because you start asking a lot of questions about if it is your own fault, and if you are strange, etc.

How do you cope with this disorder?

It is very hard on a daily basis to be in a normal school and listen to the teachers, while you are trying to ignore all the triggers. Also the family life is very hard to struggle with because if you think getting triggered on a normal basis is hard, you should try being triggered by someone you care about.
Some days are good and some days are bad. That is pretty much how I cope with it. Sometimes you just need a break from the life and people. And then you have to take one day at a time and really be patient with yourself and try to count to ten at least 30 times a day.

Are your family and friends supportive?

It's only the closest part of my family who know about Misophonia, and they are being very supportive. I'm not sure how I feel about telling others, because I think that it is seen as a weakness and I'm afraid how people would react and think.

Are you afraid to confront a person when they are triggering you?

I'm very afraid to confront people who are triggering me, because I don't want them to look at me and think that I am annoying, so I don't confront people.

If a person does not respect your condition, how do you react?

I get upset and sad, because then they know that they are hurting me and suddenly it's on purpose.

Do you have other disorders that worsen your Misophonia?

No.

Do you think the name suits the disorder? Why? Why not?

I think that it's a fine name. Actually I'm just glad that there is a name for it that I know and that other people, in the same situation know.

Are you on any drugs that do or do not help (antidepressants, anti- psychotics, etc.)?

No, and I have never tried any.

What do you think could be done to raise awareness?

I really don't know. If I knew I would probably already be doing it, but at this moment, where I'm too scared to even tell my family, how could I tell the world?

Explain the reaction when faced with a trigger:

My stomach hurts. My concentration is 110% focused on the

trigger noise, and I cannot get it away from there. I'm starting to feel the tears in my eyes and just try to hold them back. I get the feeling of sadness, anger, and I want to hit someone (myself basically). There comes a time where I no longer can stay in the situation and in the room and then I have to leave. If I don't leave I can just sit and wait for the noise to go away, trying to not let my tears get through.

Name: Victoria

Age: 25

Sex: F

Country: England

State/Province/Territory: Northamptonshire

At what age did you start to have triggers for Misophonia?

My first serious trigger was when I was about 8 when I was staying at my aunt's house, she claimed she didn't know she was chewing in my ear though it was impossible for her not to notice the angle she was sitting at. Before this, it was very mild – I did notice all my triggers but they were almost non-existent until my aunt did this – as a result I used to get grounded and banned from things because I told people to shut up when they were eating.

What are your top 5 triggers?

Any form of food in someone's mouth – even my own

Gulping – food and liquids

Hearing mucus in someone's nose – especially when I'm eating

Whistling

Biting nails

What is worse, visual triggers or audial triggers?

All of the above plus people sliding their fingers on guitar strings, also foot tapping – worst is people shaking their feet so violently one might think their foot might fall off.

When did you learn that there was a name for your condition and other sufferers?

In February 2015 through Facebook.

How did it feel to learn that there were other people like you?

I felt relieved that I wasn't going crazy, I was told I had to go and get medical help because I was supposed to have something mentally wrong with me like some sort of lunatic because it was causing problems at home, but as soon as I found out about this in February I posted it all over Facebook to prove to certain people who won't be named that I am not the psychopath they were making me out to be.

I still can't describe how happy I am now that I can put a name to this.

How do you cope with this disorder?

I often have to remove myself from the situation before I get the compulsive urge to punch someone. I also have to excuse myself from other people's houses as soon as possible so I don't do or say something that I will end up regretting.

Are your family and friends supportive?

No, they all think I'm still crazy and that I am using this to cause arguments.

Are you afraid to confront a person when they are trigger-

ing you?

I've had certain people tell me that I would get my face slapped if I did.

If a person does not respect your condition, how do you react?

Unfortunately, I have to bite my tongue in most situations, other people I will excuse myself and politely explain why I feel uncomfortable, it's their choice how they want to take that.

Do you have other disorders that worsen your Misophonia?

Severe depression.

Do you think the name suits the disorder? Why? Why not?

Well it does translate to hatred of noise, so yeah I suppose it does.

Are you on any drugs that do or do not help (antidepressants, anti- psychotics, etc.)?

No.

What do you think could be done to raise awareness?

I think there should be more charities and events and stuff to not only raise awareness but to also help provide the right support for those who don't have it at home, a good example would be a weekly meeting in a local library or have a charity café of sorts.

Explain the reaction when faced with a trigger:

The reaction I have is to punch someone so hard they think twice before setting my trigger off again, the worse the trigger is the worse my fight and flight is. Other than telling people to shut up as a child I have only ever lashed out once (verbally thankfully) asking the person to spit their gum out as they were chewing in my ear (not my aunt this time), I was in the middle of an exam at the time, so I had to really bite my tongue hard to not get up and lamp them one.

Name: Jami Blackwell

Age: 51

Sex: F

Country: USA

State/Province/Territory: Arkansas

At what age did you start to have triggers for Misophonia?
9

What are your top 5 triggers?
Gum cracking, sniffing, smacking, tapping, whistling, and throbbing bass (sorry, there's 6)

What is worse, visual triggers or audial triggers?
Audial.

When did you learn that there was a name for your condition and other sufferers?
About two and a half years ago.

How did it feel to learn that there were other people like you?
I felt relief and validation.

How do you cope with this disorder?
Mostly by avoidance or covering it with a louder noise like my

big fan or turn up the TV.

Are your family and friends supportive?

My husband and kids are. Growing up, I was just called crazy.

Are you afraid to confront a person when they are triggering you?

It depends on the trigger.

If a person does not respect your condition, how do you react?

I get highly irritated, but I try not to let it show and escape the situation as quickly as I can.

Do you have other disorders that worsen your Misophonia?

No.

Do you think the name suits the disorder? Why? Why not?

Yes, because it is a pretty much straightforward definition.

Are you on any drugs that do or do not help (antidepressants, anti- psychotics, etc.)?

I take no drugs for Misophonia.

What do you think could be done to raise awareness?

I am not sure. Maybe some documentaries or quick ads about it on TV...

Explain the reaction when faced with a trigger:

I pretty much go to instant rage... Especially if it is a rudeness thing. It isn't necessary for one to play his bass so loudly that the siding on my house vibrates. It isn't necessary for one to let his child play the drums on the chairs at church in the middle of church services. Stuff like that is just plain rude and causes instant rage. I leave the situation. It is still bad, but not quite so bad, if the trigger isn't such an outright rudeness thing.

Name: Senta K Baker

Age: 59.9

Sex: Female

Country: USA

State/Province/Territory: Indiana

At what age did you start to have triggers for Misophonia?
15

What are your top 5 triggers?
Gum chewing, lip smacking, sniffling, eating with mouth open, and chomping ice.

What is worse, visual triggers or audial triggers?
Both have the same effect on me.

When did you learn that there was a name for your condition and other sufferers?
Two years ago while watching 60 minutes TV Show.
How did it feel to learn that there were other people like you?
Started searching the Internet when I learned there was a name and found the Facebook group.

How do you cope with this disorder?
I flee, I remove myself and have recently begun using headphones.

Are your family and friends supportive?

I hid this from all of my friends until a couple of years ago I told my boss and sometimes I feel like that was a mistake. My two girls both suffer from it but on different levels and my granddaughter (3) also suffers from it by my daughter is in denial.

Are you afraid to confront a person when they are triggering you?

I so want to lash out but I just remove myself.

If a person does not respect your condition, how do you react?

My second husband was horrible, knew chomping ice set me over the edge and he was mean about it, so I would remove myself.

Do you have other disorders that worsen your Misophonia?

Not that I'm aware of.

Do you think the name suits the disorder? Why? Why not?

I haven't really thought about it either way, I'm just happy there is a name for it.

Are you on any drugs that do or do not help (antidepressants, anti- psychotics, etc.)?

I do take Xanax when I get overly anxious and it helps a bit.

What do you think could be done to raise awareness?
PSA, news articles that Joe Public would see not just scholarly journals.

Explain the reaction when faced with a trigger noise:
This past weekend I was shopping in a local drug store and there was a woman who was chewing her gum like there was no tomorrow, could almost see her molars. So I kept dodging her throughout the entire store even though I was ready to check out I had to make sure I wasn't in earshot or a visual. Waited until she checked out and then made my way, but then the gal at the counter was eating chips I just about died. Hoping to get a survey later from the store so I could complain about employees eating while waiting on customers.

Name: Alkisti Karakoli

Age: 39

Sex: F

Country: Greece

State/Province/Territory: Athens

At what age did you start to have triggers for Misophonia?
Around puberty.

What are your top 5 triggers?
People chewing with their mouth open. Lip smacking. Teeth sucking. Gulping while drinking. Pigeons. High pitched women's voices with long vowels and whistling 's' letters.

What is worse, visual triggers or audial triggers?
Audial.

When did you learn that there was a name for your condition and other sufferers?
A few years ago (2 or 3) I read an article about it on the Internet.
How did it feel to learn that there were other people like you?
It was a huge relief. I always thought I was just being weird about it and couldn't really understand why I was reacting so badly. That is, when the trigger sound stopped.

How do you cope with this disorder?

I am honest to the ones triggering me when I think they will understand. Otherwise I try to leave the area or cover my ears. I also avoid going to places like the cinema.

I haven't found a solution about the pigeon problem.

Are your family and friends supportive?

Some of them are and some of them aren't. There are also those that seem to understand me when I explain my situation but still trigger me, as they don't realize the sounds they produce.

Are you afraid to confront a person when they are triggering you?

When the trigger is 'on', I can't say I am able to have a conversation about it. I am just mad. I avoid confrontation since I know I will regret my rage afterwards. Sometimes, I can't hold it, though.

If a person does not respect your condition, how do you react?

It depends. If it's a random person I just go away or avoid people like that in general.

If it's someone close to me (like my father –it's not that he does not respect my condition, he falls in the category of people that do not realize the sounds they make) I try to find ways to be around him. Like having the TV on while we eat together, or leave the area when he has a snack etc.

Do you have other disorders that worsen your Misophonia?
No, I don't think I do.

Do you think the name suits the disorder? Why? Why not?
Not really. Since it's of Greek origin, the definition of the combined words is "hatred of voice" and that is not accurate for sounds other than voices.

Are you on any drugs that do or do not help (antidepressants, anti- psychotics, etc.)?
No.

What do you think could be done to raise awareness?
I think we need a medical proof that something we can't help is wrong with us. Otherwise, when I think about it, I understand it's really difficult for people not experiencing this to understand we are not some kind of angered freaks.

Explain the reaction when faced with a trigger:
When the trigger starts, I feel my brain is searching the area to hear the sound again. Is it there? Is it not there? Do I hear something? When it does, it locks on that direction. Then it's

almost all I can hear. The expression that comes to my mind about this is "target fixation" (I got that from motorcycle riding but it fits). After that I split in two. One part of me is looking for ways to avoid the sound and the other wants to keep hearing it...it's like a part of me wants to get annoyed... and angry... and furious. I grit my teeth and make fists with my hands. Sometimes I bang the desk in front of me (if there is a desk) before realizing I'm doing it. I want to attack the source and scream. I glance angrily, I feel... possessed. My breathing changes and I really hate the source.

When the source is someone I love, I feel so very sorry afterwards. The guilt makes me sad. Makes me cry. Who am I? What is that?

I think I've made some progress though. After experiencing this rage and guilt so many times in my life, I know what's coming then the trigger starts, so I usually choose the 'flight' solution. When I stay and try to endure it... sometimes the 'magnitude' of an incident can still surprise me. So, nope, it's not really me. But it's something I have.

Name: Ella Orr

Sex: Female

At what age did you start to have triggers for Misophonia?

I think I was about 7 or 8. I was cuddling up against my mum on the sofa, and she started to eat a banana sandwich. I remember feeling really bothered by the sound.

What are your top 5 triggers?

Wet mouth noises of all kinds, even the merest sound when someone parts their lips.

Chewing, visual and auditory - worst when open-mouthed, but still pretty bad when closed-mouthed.

Crunching.

Throat clearing.

Audible breathing through nose (especially when there is a whistling sound.)

What is worse, visual triggers or audial triggers?

Auditory triggers.

When did you learn that there was a name for your condition and other sufferers?

In my late 20s. I was curled up in bed, crying my eyes out about having to go for dinner with some relatives who were terrible about eating with their mouths open. My husband was so concerned he googled it, and came and told me about what he found.

How did it feel to learn that there were other people like you?

It was a massive relief, like a huge burden lifted from my shoulders. Beforehand I thought I was out of order for getting so annoyed. I'd beat myself up for being unreasonable and too easily irritated. I thought I was being stupid, and that I was just an unpleasant person, or maybe slightly mad. When I read about the disorder online, I started crying again – seeing people articulating the exact same things that went on in my head, with the same triggers and reactions, reassured me that it wasn't just me, and that there was actually a reason for my behaviour.

How do you cope with this disorder?

I wear earplugs at night. I listen to loud music using earphones whenever I'm on public transport. At work, if someone near me starts eating, I try and close off the nearest ear by making it look like I'm leaning on my hand, or I'll nip out to the toilets, or to the kitchen. Basically, I cope by blocking out or running away whenever it's possible.

Are your family and friends supportive?

My husband is incredibly supportive. I have also told a couple of my closest, most open-minded friends, and my mum. They

are all good about it. Other than that, I don't tell people. I tried
for a while, but I found that after spending so much of my life
bottling up the anger and keeping the suffering inside, I'm not
good at talking about it.

Are you afraid to confront a person when they are triggering
you?

Yes. I very rarely do this. I still see it as being my problem
rather than theirs. I fear coming across as whiny, irritable. I
can't fully explain to them how it makes me feel.

**If a person does not respect your condition, how do you
react?**

Mostly I consider it my fault for not explaining it properly.
Sometimes, after I have tried, the person will seem sympathetic
and interested and understanding – but their eating habits
don't change. I can't blame them for forgetting.

**Do you have other disorders that worsen your Misopho-
nia?**

I don't think so.

Do you think the name suits the disorder? Why? Why not?

As a literal description, it's fine. I'm wary about making it come
across as a phobia though.

Are you on any drugs that do or do not help (antidepres-

sants, anti psychotics, etc.)?

No. I tried going to the doctor twice. The first time I was referred to an audiologist, whose first words to me were "So, you... hear sounds too loudly?" At which point I wrote the entire attempt off. The second time, I was referred to the mental health team, who determined that there was nothing they could do about it. The only thing I have found that does help at all is alcohol. Obviously that's not a recommendation! But when I'm out and have had a few drinks, I do find that I'm less sensitive.

What do you think could be done to raise awareness?

I really don't know. If there was some comparison we could make – non- sufferers can't empathise if they have no way of relating. My husband describes it like being able to hear pain. It's difficult to get people to care about something so utterly unfathomable.

Explain the reaction when faced with a trigger:

The second I hear the tiniest trigger sounds, it's as if my entire concentration involuntarily latches on and focuses in on it. I always try to look outwardly normal, but a close observer might see that I'm gritting my teeth, pursing my lips, twitching my foot, scratching my arm... these are all signs that internally, I'm absolutely losing it. If I can't escape it, for example at a dinner table, my heart rate increases, my stomach drops, my head spins. It's an intense level of agitation and discomfort. Most of all, it's an overwhelming feeling of anger, of rage. If I look up and see a person eating their food with their mouth open, for that moment right there, I passionately hate them. In my head, I'll be screaming. I often think I would genuinely prefer physical pain. I rage against the person causing the trigger to a ridiculous degree. But – as soon as I'm free of the situation and the trigger is gone, all of those feelings disappear with it, and are replaced with crippling shame. I'll feel ridiculous, mean, crazy. I'll think about my actions in trying to deal with it, like covering my ears, beating up my computer mouse to drown it out, sitting as far as humanly possible away from everyone else at the table – and they'll feel stupidly obvious. Even though at the time, I couldn't have cared less about my actions looking weird to other people. When it's happening, I want the offender to notice me, to know I despise them, so they will just stop. Once the situation is over, I immediately feel terrible and full of regret and shame. It's like being temporarily mad.

Name: Lauren Fletcher

Age: 32

Sex: Female

Country: USA

State/Province/Territory: Tennessee

At what age did you start to have triggers for Misophonia?

The earliest I remember is around age 10.

What are your top 5 triggers?

The sound of someone chewing, especially crunchy foods; gum chewing or popping; smacking or slurping; repetitive coughing, nasal sounds or open-mouth breathing; repetitive clicking or tapping sounds.

What is worse, visual triggers or audial triggers?

Audial.

When did you learn that there was a name for your condition and other sufferers?

About a year ago. Until then, I thought there was something profoundly wrong with just me.

How did it feel to learn that there were other people like you?

I felt relieved. I stumbled across articles and Kelly Ripa's ABC interview via Pinterest, and started crying at my work desk. My therapist had been suggesting that perhaps the sound sensitivity was rooted in my eating disorder or PTSD; she had never heard of Misophonia until after I told her about the articles I'd read.

How do you cope with this disorder?

I internalize a lot. I wear earplugs when I'm in the car with my husband so I don't hear him breathing or making noises. I avoid places where I know there will be triggers. I give myself time limits in meetings so I know that I don't have to endure pen clicking or mint chewing for an extended amount of time. I keep the door closed to my office, and keep the fan on and earbuds in so I don't hear people walking by, eating or popping their gum. I wear ear plugs to the movie theatre, during dinner with my family, on planes or really any place where someone could be eating or making trigger sounds.

Are your family and friends supportive?

Somewhat. Though I've told my parents and husband about the disorder, they seem relatively oblivious to the sounds they make that bother me. My best friend does a good job of being cognizant regarding my triggers.

Are you afraid to confront a person when they are triggering you?

Yes.

If a person does not respect your condition, how do you react?

I internalize and stay away from them.

Do you have other disorders that worsen your Misophonia?

I have social anxiety disorder and obsessive-compulsive personality disorder. I'm not sure if they worsen the Misophonia, or vice versa, or if one is the result of the other. I would love to know.

Do you think the name suits the disorder? Why? Why not?

I understand the scientific significance of the name, but I'm not sure the general public would hear or read it and know that it involves hearing and/or anger. Sometimes I think the word "audio" should be included somewhere, since people usually associate that with hearing more so than the "-phonia" suffix.

Are you on any drugs that do or do not help (antidepressants, anti- psychotics, etc)?

I take Lexapro for anxiety, which has helped some. I also take Xanax periodically, especially when I'm around my triggers, which lessens the impact.

What do you think could be done to raise awareness?

There needs to be active discussion in the medical/psychological community about adding this disorder to the DSM. There need to be articles in medical and health journals. More people with the disorder

need to start speaking out about what they live with. Audiologists and psychotherapists need to start establishing relationships with each other to co-treat their patients.

Explain the reaction when faced with a trigger:

I get tunnel vision – I can't focus on anything else but that noise. Even when it's not actively happening, I am bracing myself for when it will, which increases my anxiety. When I hear the noise, the reaction in my body is the same as if I've been hit or physically injured; I tense up and feel a burning sensation in my stomach. I have the overwhelming need to run away, but the rational part of me makes me stay where I am because I know it's just a noise. I find myself giving dirty looks or exasperated stares towards the person making the noise. I am snippy with my words and my tone. I clinch my fists and try not to make eye contact with the trigger person. I think about hitting them or yelling at them to stop making the sound.

Name: Ashley

Age: 31

Sex: Female

Country: USA

State/Province/Territory: Louisiana

At what age did you start to have triggers for Misophonia?
6-7 years old.

What are your top 5 triggers?
Gum popping, food smacking/crunching, constant throat clearing, coughing, open-mouth eating.

What is worse, visual triggers or audial triggers?
Audial.

When did you learn that there was a name for your condition and other sufferers?
2012, approximately.

How did it feel to learn that there were other people like you?
It was a huge relief. It made me feel hopeful that I could overcome this disorder.

How do you cope with this disorder?

I have a strong 'flight' response. I leave if I can. If not, I just try my best to go to my 'happy place' and tell myself that it will be over eventually.

Are your family and friends supportive?
My fiancé is super supportive. He really tries to eat quietly and to make noise when other people aren't. My parents are trying to understand, but they will slip sometimes and get annoyed when I have to leave during a meal.

Are you afraid to confront a person when they are triggering you?
Yes, I have had some negative experiences when trying to be honest about the condition. I've heard responses like 'how dare you judge how I eat?' or 'you're making me feel self-conscious.'

If a person does not respect your condition, how do you react?
I refuse to be around them if I don't need to while eating.

Do you have other disorders that worsen your Misophonia?
I suffer from anxiety, but I truly feel like the Misophonia is the same no matter how I am feeling.

Do you think the name suits the disorder? Why? Why not?
I think it's perfect. I absolutely hate some sounds.

Are you on any drugs that do or do not help (antidepressants, anti- psychotics, etc.)?

No.

What do you think could be done to raise awareness?

More doctors need to specialize in the disease. People won't take it seriously unless they feel like it's a real condition.

Explain the reaction when faced with a trigger:

At first I'm in shock. I'm shocked that a person cannot control their actions/noises and I feel personally offended. I will usually stare at the person, if I can without them noticing. Then I'm disgusted and I will get angry. Some people can tell that I'm angry because I will become quiet and I will start to fidget. Then the panic (or flight) response happens. If I can, I will leave immediately. Then I usually feel guilty.

Name: Vera

Age: 24

Sex: F

Country: Canada

State/Province/Territory: Ontario

At what age did you start to have triggers for Misophonia?

I am not 100% sure but it was definitely between the ages of 7-10.

What are your top 5 triggers?

My triggers: When my mother says the letter S, and then visual with her is pointing or talking with hands type thing. My brother, it's his coughing, sniffling (throat noises) and visual it's when he shuffles his feet or wiggles his toes (leg movements). Just recently my BF started to trigger me and for him it's his throat noises also... but, nothing else just yet.

What is worse, visual triggers or audial triggers?

They are both equally as annoying. For me it's been audial. I don't have many visual triggers but if I did I would personally get more bothered by the visuals. Noises there are headphones or sound blockers but for visuals you literally just have to look away or leave the room.

When did you learn that there was a name for your condi-

tion and other sufferers?

Probably a year or two ago... I think my dad might have mentioned it before. But I hadn't really looked into it until this year. There's a lot more awareness and people coming out just these past 2 years alone.

How did it feel to learn that there were other people like you?

Umm... I felt like finally there are people I can talk to that will just get it. I have super supportive friends and family, but it feels great to know people just get it. It's also very hopeful and helpful learning people's experiences and coping mechanism.

How do you cope with this disorder?

Counting my blessing my family and friends are willing to understand and compromise. My Misophonia is only with certain people also, which has made the case less severe. HEADPHONES and SOOTHING SOUNDS or just MUSIC are key to life with Misophonia. I also try and maintain a positive attitude, good eating habits, good exercise habits etc. I don't know if it helps but what I do know is when I am stressed my triggers are x10.   Are your family and friends supportive?

Yes, they try the best they can.

Are you afraid to confront a person when they are triggering you?

No, that's the last thing I am afraid of. As terrible as this sounds if I didn't have control over my stress and anxiety, I'd be smacking everyone. But I politely tell them to stop or I plug myself into headphones.

If a person does not respect your condition, how do you react?
I've never encountered that just yet, my triggers aren't with random strangers. But I would just find them to be ignorant.

Do you have other disorders that worsen your Misophonia?
I don't think so... Stress is what really gets me. If I have a nice relaxing day my triggers are pretty under control but if it's been stressful it's like a crapshoot.

Do you think the name suits the disorder? Why? Why not?
Yeah... I think so.

Are you on any drugs that do or do not help (antidepressants, anti- psychotics, etc.)?
As a kid I was on medications (forget the names). But my parents took me off of it because it made me zombie-like. I am a Medical Marijuana patient now, and it's helped me relax my muscle spasm and virtually no reaction because I am so calm. I also eat very very well, use meditation as a muscle relaxation and staying positive. Anti-depressants and so on, if they work for you that is fine. For me I was never depressed or anything just suffer from Misophonia. So what those drugs did is take my mind and kept the Misophonia... counter-productive.

What do you think could be done to raise awareness?

I think people should be going to offices, schools etc., where people have to work and deal with this condition in everyday life. It educates the person suffering and the people around them.

Explain the reaction when faced with a trigger:

I feel anger, sadness and stress. But I constantly have to remind myself it's not them nor me it's the Misophonia Monster.

Name: Sharon Mousel

Age: 19

Sex: Female

At what age did you start to have triggers for Misophonia?
10.

What are your top 5 triggers?
"S" sounds
Foot tapping Chewing/gulping/smacking Slurping
Fork hitting teeth

What is worse, visual triggers or audial triggers?
Audial.

When did you learn that there was a name for your condition and other sufferers?
Age 15.

How did it feel to learn that there were other people like you?
It felt amazing. It kind of made Misophonia valid to me.

How do you cope with this disorder?
I use earplugs and headphones. I took magnesium for a little bit, but it didn't work out for me.

Are your family and friends supportive?

Yes.

Are you afraid to confront a person when they are triggering you?

No. I'm not afraid, but I don't confront people if they are triggering me, I just leave if I can. The reason why is because I know asking someone, "Please stop breathing" or "Please stop eating like a pig" will seem very irrational to someone. Unless I'm wearing my bracelet that says "Misophonia Awareness", I'd show it to them and just bring up a conversation about it, and tell them I have it.

If a person does not respect your condition, how do you react?

Fortunately, I haven't encountered someone I don't know who disrespected my condition. Back in the day though, my dad and my aunt were not supportive of my condition, and since I couldn't tell them what I had—because I didn't know—they thought I was being bratty and kept triggering me.

Do you have other disorders that worsen your Misophonia?

Not that I know of.

Do you think the name suits the disorder? Why? Why not?

While "Misophonia" is the more popular name (and I use it

a lot), I do prefer "Selective Sound Sensitivity Syndrome" if I was to introduce it to someone I've never met before. It sounds more professional, I think. I would also mention the term "Misophonia" and that it is more popularly known as that.

Are you on any drugs that do or do not help (antidepressants, anti- psychotics, etc.)?
No.

What do you think could be done to raise awareness?
I put on a T-shirt campaign and many of my family members bought a shirt. I hope it spreads awareness. I think bracelets are a more efficient way to spread awareness, however. I also did a research report on it for a class, so my teacher became aware of it. I also tell my teachers ahead of time that I may need to wear headphones during class, and I would explain I have Misophonia.

Explain the reaction when faced with a trigger:
At first, it's anxiety, but that's only if I know someone is going to, say, slurp a cup of coffee in front of me. Next, it's anger. Extreme anger. And I sometimes hit something if it's really bad. When it's all said and done, I feel tired and slightly moody.

Name: Victoria MacNeil-LeBlanc

Age: 17

Sex: Female

Country: Canada

State/Province/Territory: Ontario (Toronto)

At what age did you start to have triggers for Misophonia?

Around age 10 or so, but I do have one memory of reacting very negatively to my father whistling when I was 6 or 7 years old.

What are your top 5 triggers?

Gum and general open mouthed chewing, nail biting, loud breathing, finger and foot tapping, and nail picking.

What is worse, visual triggers or audial triggers?

Audial triggers, but I am affected by visual triggers as well.

When did you learn that there was a name for your condition and other sufferers?

I read about it in a "weird personality quirks that are actually medical conditions" article online (on Cracked) when I was 15 years old, in May 2013.

How did it feel to learn that there were other people like you?

It felt great to learn that I'm not a rude, controlling person, and

I'm not the only one. My parents thought that I was a controlling brat, it was nice to learn that my behaviour had an explanation and was not inappropriate.

How do you cope with this disorder?

Asking my parents/friends to stop triggering me, always having earplugs/headphones with me, avoiding specific people/events that trigger me.

Are your family and friends supportive?

Mostly. My dad can get pretty angry sometimes when I ask him to stop triggering me, especially when it's a visual trigger, but I know that, ultimately, he wants me to be happy and healthy. My mom is supportive, but gets mad if I "sound angry" when I ask her to stop triggering me. Otherwise, they're nice and supportive, probably around 97% of the time. My best friend is the only other person who knows, and she's supportive.

Are you afraid to confront a person when they are triggering you?

Yes, I've never confronted anyone except for my parents and best friend, and probably never would. I'm very shy.

If a person does not respect your condition, how do you react?

With anger internally, but externally I try to remain calm and respond in a sophisticated, intelligent way, in an attempt to almost shame them for their ignorance and inability to respect invisible diseases/disorders.

Do you have other disorders that worsen your Misophonia?
No. I have OCD and a few other issues but I don't believe that any of them make my Misophonia any worse.

Do you think the name suits the disorder? Why? Why not?
Yes, I do. I only wish that Misophonia didn't literally mean hatred of sounds, because saying I have the hatred of sounds when trying to explain my visual triggers is very awkward and nearly impossible to explain.

Are you on any drugs that do or do not help (antidepressants, anti- psychotics, etc.)?
I'm not on any drugs, because I can't do blood tests.

What do you think could be done to raise awareness?
The books and movies/documentaries planned are a great start. The websites are also good for educating the masses, and I'm a writer for a
website (misophonia4s.weebly.com) about Misophonia. I'd also like to see Misophonia discussed more often on the radio/TV, but it must be done with respect. I've heard a local radio station (104.5 Chum FM) make fun of Misophonia, purposely trig-

gering a woman by making loud chewing/ slurping noises into the microphone while she tried to explain it to the DJ. It was disgusting and hurtful, and probably set the Misophonia movement back a few years by making thousands of listeners think that it's just a joke. So, if Misophonia could be addressed with respect by the media that would be great. If I ever get rich, I'm going to put out commercials and advertisements about Misophonia, seriously.

Explain the reaction when faced with a trigger:
I feel immediate disgust and anger... I need it to stop, somehow. If it's a parent or friend, I ask them to stop. I try to be respectful and polite but it often comes out sounding rude because I'm angry. A lot of Misophonia sufferers have issues with controlling their anger when they're being subjected to a trigger, but few non-sufferers understand this and take offense. If it's someone I can't talk to, I try to obstruct my hearing somehow, using earplugs or headphones. If I can leave, I do leave. However, most of the time, I'm triggered during class, so I can't leave. If I have to hear a trigger for too long, I get very overwhelmed and feel like crying. I've never actually cried, but I've come very close. Sometimes, to distract myself, I pinch my hand or arm. Never too hard, rarely ever hard enough to even leave a mark. It's always just hard enough to draw my attention to the physical sensation, which can be very relieving compared to hearing a trigger.

Name: Cathy Bacchus

Age: 57

Sex: Female

Country: Canada

State/Province/Territory: British Columbia (Vernon)

At what age did you start to have triggers for Misophonia?
About 9 or 10.

What are your top 5 triggers?
Gum chewing (visual and sound), crunchy or mouth noises with food, tapping, bass or music or voice sounds (i.e. cars/neighbours).

What is worse, visual triggers or audial triggers?
Audial.

When did you learn that there was a name for your condition and other sufferers?
About 2006 or 2007.

How did it feel to learn that there were other people like you?
Didn't feel as crazy or alone.

How do you cope with this disorder?

Avoidance most of the time, stay inside my home, use headphones, noise machines, fans, or earplugs.

Are your family and friends supportive?

When I was younger or before I knew – No. Marriage break up, etc. Some friends are supportive but do not understand.

Are you afraid to confront a person when they are triggering you?

Yes.

If a person does not respect your condition, how do you react?

Anxiety, want to flee. If not, anger inside or self-harm.

Do you have other disorders that worsen your Misophonia?

Yes, anxiety, depression, OCD.

Do you think the name suits the disorder?

Why? Why not?

No, because I think it's more of a sensitivity-pain. It gives me a physical reaction, which causes fear, which is not necessarily a hatred of sounds – it makes my body sick.

Are you on any drugs that do or do not help (antidepressants, anti- psychotics, etc.)?

Fluoxetine, Dexedrine, Diazepam, etc. but they don't take away the sensitivity to sound or visual triggers.

What do you think could be done to raise awareness?

Doctors or counsellors to believe in us and do more research.

Explain the reaction when faced with a trigger:

I feel sick, my body twitches, and I want to run away. I get tearful and feel like I am going to scream or explode in anger. I have caused self-harm to try and alleviate the strong feelings, or used drugs to get some sleep.

Name: Martin

Age: 22

Country: México

State/Province/Territory: Jalisco/Guadalajara

At what age did you start to have triggers for Misophonia?
8-9

What are your top 5 triggers?
Chewing gum

Chips cracking

Popping gum

Hearing my family members softly singing Hearing my neighbors music

What is worse, visual triggers or audial triggers?
The same, but the audial are more frequent on my daily life.

When did you learn that there was a name for your condition and other sufferers?
About June or July of 2014 in a website called 9gag.com, in the comments section from a post.

How did it feel to learn that there were other people like you?
It was a weight off my shoulders. It almost felt like having a

"superpower" and knew there were more people with it that can help you to control it.

How do you cope with this disorder?

I try to live day by day the most normally possible, always carrying my earbuds and of course I have to eat alone (at least when I'm with my family), because for some reason I don't get mad or annoyed when I hear my friends eat.

But most important, I think the music I listen helps me a lot to calm or get rid of my rage. I listen to metal music.

Are your family and friends supportive?

Most of the time, they try to no eat anything when I'm near to them.

Are you afraid to confront a person when they are triggering you?

Not really. Usually I'm a peaceful person and I would prefer to walk away.

If a person does not respect your condition, how do you react?

I don't really know, because only my family knows that I have it.

Do you have other disorders that worsen your Misophonia?

No.

Do you think the name suits the disorder? Why? Why not?
No, because I think there is not enough medical studies to tell this must be a disorder.

Are you on any drugs that do or do not help (antidepressants, anti- psychotics, etc.)?
No.

What do you think could be done to raise awareness?
Make a viral campaign.

Explain the reaction when faced with a trigger:
First of all when I notice the trigger, all my senses begin to sharp and unconsciously focus on the sound. Then I have to quickly see the environment I'm on, if I can walk away, I took that option, if not, I have to take out my earbuds and begin to listen my music until I can get the trigger out of my head. If for any reason I don't have my earbuds, or just can't use them for being in my job or something serious, I turn my face into a "I'm going to punch you so f*cking hard if you don't stop" looking face and then I begin to stare the person who is making the trigger until they get I'm mad. If that doesn't work I use my last resort... begin to mimic the sounds or the trigger moves that the person is making.

And by the way, fortunately I haven't reached the point that I want to punch someone for trigger me with misophonia related things, in the worst-case scenario I just think that I would scream to the person to stop doing the trigger.

How To Cope

How do you cope with a disorder that most of the world, including doctors and researchers, don't know exists? In my experience, sufferers deal with this with great difficulty. I've heard of people trying radical methods to help cope with Misophonia. Since it's so debilitating, many are willing to try absolutely anything to combat the negative aspects of the disorder. This chapter will discuss methods that have been used by people with Misophonia, my own personal experience, as well as any research or medical claims that back up a method, where available. Please understand that, while frustrating, there is currently no official cure for Misophonia. These methods may help one person and not another. Your best defense against Misophonia is to use trial and error and respect your journey to find peace of mind.

I used to think that avoidance was the best way to stay away from triggers. But, I eventually realized that this was counterintuitive. When "missing out" on important events and socialization, I began to realize that this made me anxious and depressed. Then, I would be triggered more if I happened to be in the situation. Obviously this isn't what we want to happen. Instead, it's important that we practice mindfullness and are aware of our limits but willing and ready to compromise, try, and live a full life despite our limitations and our disorder.

Misophonia is not a life sentence.

There's no question that Misophonia changes the lives of those who suffer from it. It also changes the lives of parents, siblings, friends, and romantic partners. This doesn't mean that you need to hide out for your entire life. Sure, it's hard to live with, but life is still possible with these complications. With a few adjustments, you can have a normal, fulfilling life.

You may have to change what your idea of "normal" is to match your needs. After all, life is about what you make it. Stop thinking of Misophonia as something that has "happened to you" and start thinking about it as an interesting part of you. I know that can be hard to consider. After all, it sucks. But, think of it this way - this is a part of who you are, for better or worse.

Susan Nesbit, O.T. has come up with a "Sensory Diet". This diet is usually used to help SPD sufferers. However, if Misophonia is a part of the SPD spectrum, this may be very helpful. Personally I find the information on sensory regulation to be very helpful. The best part of this is that there are little to no negative side effects. If something does not work simply stop doing it. I have been using information from this diet for the past four months and I feel more energetic and better equip to handle triggers as they come. Life isn't as bleak as it used to be.

If you find trouble coming up with ways to use the Sensory Diet, but find some of it to be beneficial you may want to look into finding an Occupational Therapist in your area. An

O.T. would be able to personalize a regulation program for your needs, and may be able to help you better adjust to the disorder.

A printable version of the Sensory Diet can be found at misophoniainternational.com/sensory-diet-by-susan-nesbit-o-t/

It is important to note that this Sensory Diet was created for SOR (Sensory Over-Responsivity). However, there is no reason to believe that the Sensory Diet cannot help alleviate sympoms of what we now call "Misophonia". Regardless of the names involved, each and every person is entirely different. What works for your sister may have little to no impact on you. It is important that you learn your own system, and for this reason, I reccomend you consult with an O.T. that at least has a working knowledge of SPD or other Sensory related disorders. Trust yourself above all. You are the one who spends the most time inside your head and therefore you are the one who has a great deal of the answers for yourself.

Please note that the following guide is not meant to be used in place of consulting with a doctor or an O.T. There is little information about Misophonia, but still, you should alert your doctor as to your condition and your progresses. Please do not be afraid to tell your doctor that you're having a problem. If you are uncomfortable with your doctor, or feel as though he or she isn't taking you seriously, change doctors. It is of the utmost importance that you have the doctor that is right for you.

Some doctors are simply not the right match for the patient. This is not to say that they are not a good doctor, it is merely a reflection of your one on one relationship. Don't be afraid to ask questions and to shop around. Your health is of the utmost importance. Never forget that.

Sensory Diet for Teenagers and Adults
Susan Nesbit, M.S., OT/L, OT (C)

Patricia and Julia Wilbarger coined the term sensory diet. Persons with sensory over-responsivity (SOR) – a subtype of sensory processing disorders (SPD) – use sensory diets to stay calm, energized, and organized. Sensory diets are used for SOR in many sensory channels, including the auditory (sounds), the visual (sights), the tactile (touch), and the olfactory (smells). Note: The term SPD often is used interchangeably with SOR, including auditory over-responsivity. To be in sync with others, I used the term SPD in this document, unless the more narrow term of SOR or auditory-responsivity is needed for clarity.

Whether a sensory diet also is helpful for persons with misophonia is unclear. Sensory diets were developed to treat SOR. If the causes of misophonia are different, then a sensory diet may not be effective. Scholars have speculated that both conditions are neurologically based, and perhaps the same structures in the brain are involved. Scholars from both camps proposed that the limbic system plays a role. The limbic system controls our emotions and the fight-flight-freeze response. The amygdala filters out the unimportant and irrelevant sensory information so it does not reach the limbic system. Deep pressure and slow movement are theorized to help the amygdala act as a filter. If the amygdala plays a role in misophonia, then a sensory diet could lessen the impact of the triggers so persons can respond with less adversity to noxious sounds (triggers).

Research is needed to investigate the similarities and the differences between auditory over-responsivity and misophonia.

The Purpose of a Sensory Diet: Use a strategic mix of sensory activities to reduce meltdowns (e.g., yelling or snapping at someone) and shutdowns (withdrawing).

Definition of Sensory Dieting: Similar to eating food every few hours, the body needs to be replenished with sensory input. You may need to do a sensory diet every one-two hours. Sensory diets can be used at specific daily time periods or as needed. Choose one or more activities. Doing a sensory diet for 5-15 minutes can be helpful; however, doing a sensory diet for 30 minutes has a longer-lasting effect.

Essential Ingredients in a Sensory Diet: Proprioceptive (pressure) and vestibular (movement) inputs can be calming and organizing. Swinging is the ideal source of vestibular input. The effect in the brain from 15 minutes of swinging is reported to last up to eight hours. Other types of sensory input affect the brain for one-to-two hours. Some experts recommend swinging for at least 15 minutes, 2 times per day (e.g., early morning and late afternoon). Because a swing hung from one hook can be moved at varying speeds (e.g., fast) and in more directions, using a swing hung from a single hook gives more intense and longer-lasting input than a swing hung from two hooks. Important points: Slow, linear, and rhythmical movements are calming and fast, rotary, and erratic movements are excitatory.

Proprioceptive input is speculated to help integrate vestibular input. Climb and jump after swinging. Proprioceptive input can be used alone without vestibular input. Proprioceptive input is gotten through "heavy work" such as carrying books, moving furniture and vacuuming, and lifting free weights.

Proprioceptive input can be calming, energizing, and organizing. So when in doubt, use heavy work (proprioception).

Notes on Other Types of Sensory Input

Auditory (sounds) – Many persons with auditory over-responsivity or misophonia can avoid becoming overwhelmed by controlling and predicting the noxious sounds (triggers). So take some control over the environmental noises, whenever possible.

Visual (sights) – Visual input can be over-arousing for persons with auditory sensitivities. Simplify your visual field for a calming and organizing effect. Avoid clothes, towels, rugs, wall colors, etc., in colors that you find distressing. In contrast, if you feel "tuned out," add brightly colored objects to encourage visual attention.

Tactile (touch) – Tactile input can be over-arousing. Light touch can be noxious; firm touch can be calming. Avoid clothes with labels, etc., that you find distressing.

Olfactory (smells) – Odors calm, stimulate, or send a person into sensory overload. Persons with olfactory over-responsivity can become upset by something "stinky."

Precautions: Avoid using lavender products with boys who have not yet reached puberty. In several recent studies, researchers found a link with breast growth. Experts also suggest not using these products with girls because the effects are not yet known. Lavender also has precautions for adults. When applied to the skin, for example, it sometimes causes irritation.

Other oils can cause irritation when applied directly to the skin. Experiment on small patches of skin before applying oils in large quantities. Putting a few drops into a warm bath can lower the risk of skin irritation. You can use a diffuser to dispense the oils; however, this method has a less intense impact.

Women who are pregnant or breast-feeding should avoid some of the oils listed below. Some of them should be discontinued 2 weeks prior to surgery, as they can negatively interact with the anesthesia.

Explore the scents to find the ones that best meet your needs – calming (soothing) versus alerting (waking up), and to find the aromas that you prefer.

Scents that generally are calming and relaxing: Lavender, rose, rosemary, chamomile, ylang ylang, vanilla (the smell of vanilla in hot tea can make some persons nauseous), and frankincense.

Scents that generally are alerting without causing over-stimulation: Citrus – the best oils for feeling awake (e.g., bergamot, grapefruit, orange, lemon, and lime), mint (e.g., peppermint and spearmint), pine (e.g., juniper and white fur), eucalyptus, and some condiments and spices (e.g., basil, rosemary, and cinnamon).

http://www.alertprogram.com

This website has a one-page PDF handout explaining the Alert Program. You can buy a book called "How Does Your Engine Run? – A Leaders Guide to The Alert Program for Self-Regulation," written by Mary Sue Williams and Sherry Shellenberger. The program has step-by-step instructions to help you identify your level of alertness (arousal) and activities that can enable your engine to run at an optimal speed. Many therapists, teachers, and parents have taught themselves how to use the program by reading this book. The program can be used to help others or yourself.

Guidelines

1. For persons with SPD, the activities listed in this sensory diet are suggestions. The ideas are not intended to be cookbook recipes. Consider buying the book for the Alert Program to identify your level of arousal and the activities that are calming, energizing, and organizing for you. Alternatively, consult with an occupational therapist for a thorough evaluation and an individualized sensory diet.

2. Use activities based on your interests. Start with something simple and gradually move on to something more challenging.

3. Routines can be important. However, occasionally changing the routine might help you expand your interests if you desire to do so.

4. Pay attention to your mind/body. Notice when you need to cool off or calm down. Watch for signs that you are starting to relax after switching to calming activities.

5. Activities that work for you one day may not work for you on a different day. Although a sensory diet has consistencies, variations occur from day to day and moment to moment, based on the noxious stimuli that have accumulated on that day at that moment.

6. Although I listed a particular activity once, putting it into only one category – calming, energizing, or organizing – some of the activities can be used in more than one category. Heavy work (defined as pushing and pulling against resistance and carrying heavy items) can be calming, energizing, and/or organizing. Use a strategic mix of sensory activities by paying attention to your mind/body. Note: When in doubt, use heavy work (proprioception).

7. Borrowing the wisdom from the quote, "If you know one person with autism, then you know one person with autism," one can say, "If you know one person with SPD, then you know one person with SPD." In other words, all persons with SPD are unique individuals. So the sensory diet that works for one person, might not work for another person.

8. Talk with an occupational therapist regularly, when possible, to be certain the sensory diet continues to fit your sensory needs.

To Create a Strategic Mix: Sensory diets should include calming, energizing (alerting), and organizing activities to be used based on your performance. Develop an individualized sensory diet using the lists below as a guide. Use calming activities during periods of high arousal or stress and energizing activities during low periods.

Calming Activities

If you are over-stimulated, the following activities may help to calm you.

- Hugging/bear hugging with a partner
- Tightly wrapping your arms around your torso and/or crossing your legs and/or squeezing your hands together
- Cuddling with a partner or pets
- Getting a firm massage or backrub with deep/firm pressure – light touch or stroking could be alerting
- Pushing against a wall with back, buttocks, hands, head, or shoulders
- Pushing against a wall as if to move it
- Leaning forward with hands on edge of desk or table – gently pushing as if to move it; doing pushups if table is stable
- Pushing into a chair with hands on the sides; holding self above chair with both arms; doing chair pushups
- Rolling up tightly in a blanket
- Slow rocking in a sleeping bag
- Slow rocking, e.g., in a rocking chair
- Swinging with slow, linear, and rhythmical movements (e.g., on a hammock)
- Carrying books or other heavy objects across a room or up and down the stairs
- Wearing a heavy backpack (Precautions: the conservative

estimate to prevent injuries is to carry no more than 10% of your body weight, with 15-20% being less conservative estimates; use a backpack with wide and padded shoulder straps, a padded back, and a waist strap; distribute the load so it does not become bottom-heavy or top-heavy, and wear the backpack across both shoulders)

• Wearing a heavy backpack while carrying a few books

• Wearing weighted collars, pillows, or blankets (heed precautions, especially with weighted vests)

• Taking a slow walk at sunset

• Walking/strolling in a park

• Swimming laps

• Lifting free weights

• Carrying the laundry basket

• Washing windows, mirrors, or tables

• Pushing and pulling heavy items (e.g., yard work): Mowing the lawn (with a push lawn mower), raking, shoveling dirt or snow (heed safety precautions to avoid straining), and pushing firewood in a wheelbarrow

• Enjoying leisure activities (e.g., reading or listening to books on tape) in a quiet space filled with pillows for cuddling (Avoid over-stimulating visual distractions: Use dim lighting, close the drapes/shades or sit with your back to the windows, use solid-colored furniture and rugs versus patterned ones and solid-colored walls in soft or neutral colors versus patterned wallpaper in bold colors, hide clutter in bins or boxes or behind doors or curtains – e.g., hang a solid-color curtain over a bookshelf, and avoid wearing clothing in colors that you find distressing – and consider asking your loved ones, friends, and colleagues to avoid wearing clothes in colors that you find distressing)

• Watching the fish swimming in an aquarium

• Watching and listening to the flames in a bonfire or fireplace, especially a fireplace with real wood

• Listening to rain, a waterfall, and ocean waves

• Listening to a tabletop fountain or an aquarium

• Listening to quiet/soothing/relaxing music such as Mozart and Baroque music, e.g., Bach, Handel, Pachelbel, and Vivaldi

• Listening to colored noise (e.g., white, pink, and grey); however, some persons find colored noise to be irritating

• Taking a warm bath or shower, then rolling up in a large towel (avoid using towels in colors that you find distressing)

• Using calming scents such as lavender and/or rose in oils, soaps, lotions, or candles (strong scents can be alerting rather than calming, so experiment)

• Wearing compression clothing, e.g., short-sleeved and long-sleeved t-shirts, shorts, and pants

Energizing Activities

If you need to be aroused, wake up your senses by trying

some of these activities:

• Tug-of-War (pull on TheraBand tied around the door-knob of a closed door; use the strongest resistance possible)

• Pulling heavy items, e.g., suitcase or backpack on wheels

• Jumping jacks/star jumps on the floor

• Jumping on a mini-trampoline (use a backyard trampo-line if one is available)

• Jumping rope

• Bouncing on a hopper ball, exercise ball, or therapy ball (these balls come in adult sizes)

• Brisk/vigorous walking and race walking

• Hiking uphill

• Stair climbing: Race up the stairs, then go up the stairs two at a time (to cool off, walk at a normal pace down the stairs)

• Aerobics, including chair aerobics

• Calisthenics, e.g., lunges, squat jumps, sit-ups, pushups, and pull-ups

• Tumbling, e.g., cartwheels

• Swimming: Doing flips and somersaults in the water

• Swing dancing

• Spinning in rotating chair or on swing suspended from one hook

• Using playground swings or a merry-go-round (you're never too old)

• Taking a cool shower

• Using alerting scents such as citrus, mint, and/or pine in oils, soaps, lotions, or candles

Organizing Activities

These activities may calm or energize, depending on your needs. Pay attention to your body for signs that indicate your level of arousal.

• Squeezing stress balls

• Sucking, e.g., water from a squeeze bottle, a popsicle, a lifesaver

• Sucking drinkable (liquid) yogurt through a straw

• Eating healthy, crunchy foods like carrots or chewy food like jellybeans

• Chewing bubble gum

• Blowing soap bubbles

• Climbing stairs (up and down) or a ladder

• Doing pushups (on the floor from knees or toes; standing and leaning forward against a wall)

• Doing sit-ups

• Doing jumping jacks

• Tumbling and gymnastics

• Doing headstands or handstands against a wall

• Hiking, walking, or running

• Roller skating, roller blading, or ice skating

• Jumping rope

• Biking/cycling

- Horseback riding

- Stretching, including tai chi and yoga

- Lying on your stomach to read a book

- Painting the walls with plain and/or textured paints, e.g., add sand to the paint

- Pushing heavy items, e.g., shopping cart, laundry basket, or box filled with books

- Pulling heavy items, e.g., wagon filled with children, books or laundry detergent

- Vacuuming – especially when pushing the furniture out of the way!

- Taking out the rubbish/garbage/trash or hauling bags of leaves to the curb

- Creating a scrapbook: Ripping/tearing paper, using different textures, gluing (squeeze bottle) or pasting, and painting

- Coloring mandalas – begin at the center and work your way to the outside border; use colored pencils or crayons, because markers leak and destroy the experience

- Sewing, knitting, crocheting, and weaving

- Sculpting: Making things out of clay through coil or slab methods; try using a potter's wheel

- Woodworking: Sawing, gluing in dowels, pounding nails, screwing in nuts and bolts, using sandpaper to smooth the project

- Baking: Mixing the ingredients in a bowl (not using an electric mixer), and squeezing/kneading, flattening, and rolling the dough for bread or cookies

• Cooking: Pounding chicken cutlets with a food hammer and chopping vegetables

• Gardening: Digging, patting soil, pulling weeks, carrying and pouring water from a large watering can, and pouring/dumping dirt or mulch

Organizing Games and Partnership or Group Activities

• Tug-of-War

• Tennis or badminton

• Softball or baseball

• Volleyball

• Basketball

• Kickball or soccer

• Martial arts, including tae kwon do and karate

• Races, e.g., adult relay races, 5K and 10K runs, ½ and full marathons, and track

• Dancing and singing

Example of a Sensory Diet

Personalize this example. To meet your changing sensory needs, modify the activities as your needs change. Use a strategic mix of activities.

General suggestions: Take frequent movement breaks, sit on an inflatable wobble cushion, and chew crunchy foods (e.g., carrots) during daily activities that require attention and concentration. Rocking gently before bedtime can help with a sleeping problem. Try a firm self-hug after rocking.

In the morning:

• Upon awakening, massage your neck and shoulders: Gently but firmly move your fingers in small circles – start at the base of your skull and move down your neck and then out toward one shoulder and repeat toward the other shoulder - work out the knots – then stretch by hugging yourself

• Take a bath or a cool shower with alerting scents such as citrus, mint, or pine

• Use a vibrating toothbrush and/or a vibrating hairbrush

• Listen to music that you find alerting but not over-stimulating

• Eat crunchy cereal with fruit and some protein

• Take a brisk or vigorous walk or jump on a mini-trampoline

Midafternoon:

• Do aerobic exercises or jump on a mini-trampoline

• Go for a bicycle ride or do yoga

• Push a grocery cart or a stroller, depending on family needs

• Massage your feet to "reorganize"

• Listen to music that you find alerting but not over-stimulating

• Oral work – Suck liquid yogurt through a straw, eat crunchy and chewy snacks, or chew gum before and/or during activities at a desk or table

At dinnertime:

• Make a meal with mixing, chopping, pounding, and so on

• Set the table, using two hands to carry and balance a heavy but stable tray

• Eat crunchy and chewy foods

At night:

• Take a walk/stroll in a park

• Sew, sculpt clay, or make woodworking projects or scrapbooks

• Color mandalas – begin at the center and work your way to the outside border; use colored pencils or crayons

• Take a warm bath with bubbles and calming essential

oils such as lavender or rose

• Listen to quiet/soothing/relaxing music such as Mozart and Baroque music, e.g., Bach, Handel, Pachelbel, and Vivaldi

• Massage

- Susan Nesbit

Living a Healthy Lifestle

No matter the disorder, I am a firm believer that a healthy lifestyle is our first line of defense. We would not want to send soldiers into battle malnourished, tired, sluggish, and dehydrated. So, why then, does it seem perfectly okay to stuff ourselves with cakes and soda and assume that our problems aren't becoming worse because of it? After all, our bodies are only able to work with the tools that they have.

I have been struggling with Anxiety and Depression for ten years. Through that journey I have learned that the most important tool for understanding coping and our bodies, is to understand that we are beings that live lives of connectivity. Mental, physical, spiritual being are not separate things to check off our list. Where one waivers - others will soon follow. Practicing mindfulness is the first step to recognizing that you are going to be the one to make your world a better place. Whether this means donating your money to research, or simply being proactive about your health - you are the sole propietor of your body and mind.

Water Intake

It isn't a coincidence that water holds a place at the top of this list. Water is absolutely crucial for a healthy lifestyle. I never knew how dehydrated I have been for years until I started drinking an appropriate amount of water. Like a good shower, water has washed away a lot of the cloudiness from my life. Triggers aren't completely alleviated but I have more energy, am less stressed, and I feel as though the world is a brighter place. There's never an excuse not to drink enough water, ever. I swear by the practice. In order to make it feasible, I use a free iPhone app called Waterlogged to track how much water I drink daily. I don't always make my goal, and when I don't, I notice it quickly. The negative aftermath goes well into the next day. The rule I follow is to drink half your weight in ounces.

While some doctors and nutritionists have other ideas, this works for me. I feel so much better now that I drink a good amount of water every day. For example, since I am 150 lbs. right now, I drink at least 75 ounces of water a day. I usually exceed my goals by rounding up to 80 ounces. To make it easier, I measure my water in 20 oz. bottles, and then pour it into a glass. Once I'm done with the entire bottle I register it in the app.

Additionally, I have measured my teacups. Each cup of tea is 10 ounces of water. I get a lot of my water from herbal tea, which I used to hate. Remember, the feeling of thirst means you're already dehydrated. Drink water at regular intervals throughout the day. You may want to before bedtime, as a full bladder can lead to restlessness and an inability to sleep.

You may want more water depending on how you feel, or if you're very active. Listen to your body. If you're not sure about your daily intake, make sure you consult your doctor. Don't be afraid to ask questions that sound odd. It's perfectly reasonable to ask your doctor about your water intake. It's wise, even.

Diet

Misophonia may not be cured by eating right, but a lot of people who suffer from the disorder have noted that they feel much better, and are triggered less, when on a healthy and 'clean' diet. On my fridge, I have a quote taped to the front. It reads, "You are what you eat. So, don't be cheap, easy and fake". High sugar and processed diets aren't doing you any favors. This is especially true if you are already dealing with a condition as strange and discouraging as Misophonia. Perhaps eating right won't 'cure' the illness, but eating improperly leads to stress on the body, and when you're stressed, you're more likely to be triggered.

Let's not forget the added risks of this highly processed diet: cancer, diabetes, hypertension, heart disease, and many others. Beware- the modern diet hides sugar everywhere, and all of my research on health has led me to believe that all sugar is sugar, and sugar is bad. Some interesting books and documentaries highlight exactly why sugar is so deadly. Several doctors are now comparing sugar to poison and believe that sugar leads to a plethora of negatives.

In 1972, before much of the world had caught on, John Yudkin wrote a book explaining the dangers of sugar, entitled *Pure, White and Deadly*. Aside from being a university professor he was also had an M.D, PhD, and M.A. Yudkin believed that, "The consumption of sugar on top of an ordinary diet increases the risk of obesity; the consumption of sugar instead of part of an adequate diet increases the risk of nutritional deficiencies" (55). If you want to avoid sugar you must be mindful, it is in nearly every processed food, and "In the food industry, finding the bliss point for sugar in dinner products like pasta sauce would soon become passé. Products for meals were relatively easy" (Moss 103) and continue to be in these foods, and many more.

Personally, I feel much better now that I have incorporated a significant amount of vegetables, proper protein, and reduced sugar, sodium, and processed food intake considerably in my diet. It's important to believe that healthy food is not worse, or a punishment. When done right, healthy food is highly rewarding and delicious.

I would never reccomend a fad or niche diet. I'm a firm believer in nutrition being a very personal thing. It is not a one size fits all ordeal. Some people are lactose intolerant, but others aren't. I eat milk, cheese and dairy, despite certain warnings. Personally I have opted for organic options and I feel much better. But, it's up to you to determine your relationship with foods. You may want to practice mindfullness and explore what exactly is being pumped into your body at every turn.

Since there is little proof as to what exactly long-term chemical exposure, or even GMOs are going to do to the body, I believe it is important to be considerate of these factors. That does not mean that you should make choices based on conspiracy theories but simply be aware. You should try different options and see what your body thinks about it. Let your mental and physical health be your guide for what is right for you.

As for cooking, it is an important part of the daily ritual. As you can see, it is mentioned in Susan Nesbit's sensory diet. Much of modern life has become an avoidance of preparation and "busy work". But, it is these exact activities that may help us to regulate our sensory systems. As well, preparing your meals yourself gives your body the proper chance it needs to prepare for food and aids digestion.

The following documentaries talk about nutrition, especially the negative impact of sugar and processed foods in the diet. An asterisk (*) by the title indicates that it is a personal favourite of mine. Remember to always second-guess information. Who was speaking? Was it a doctor? A nutritionist? Do research studies back this up? What does MY doctor think?

Though I enjoy these documentaries they are meant to be talking points. It is important to be educated and make wise decisions when considering what is healthful.

The Documentaries are:

» Fed Up*

» Food Matters

» Fat, Sick, and Nearly Dead Supersize Me

» Forks Over Knives*

» Hungry For Change Vegucated

» Food Matters

» A Place at the Table*

Exercise

The least fun out of any of these, exercise always seems to land at the bottom of every to-do list. Aside from some gym enthusiasts, exercise is seen as some form of modern torture. I have to admit, I'm not a fan. However, I won't dispute that for some, exercise can provide an amazing high. The endorphins released will help you to deal with stress, possibly triggers, and as a bonus, you'll be sweating out the toxins that can be harmful to your body. You don't have to train for a marathon or be an Olympic swim champion to reap the benefits from exercise. Start off slowly. Thirty minutes, three times a week of a physical activity that you enjoy will get the ball rolling, and the more you do, the more you'll feel able and willing to do it. Try to make exercise fun by bringing a friend along. A friend who understands your Misophonia and who is willing to compromise will be best. You don't want to be trying to combat triggers while trying to de-stress. However, if you're already triggered, you can use exercise as a way to relieve the tension and beat out the anger. Think boxing.

If you push aside all your excuses you're left with one fact: Exercise will help to improve the overall quality of your life. When I first wrote this section I was entirely unaware of the proposed benefits from sensory diets or the role exercise can play. Since learning this I have been considering all options and trying things that may help to regulate, instead of just picking an exercise and going for it.

I like to choose things like swimming because I feel most comfortable in the water. But, I live in Canada so this can be hard in the winter. That's when I enjoy things like bowling, skating, or sledding. I'll admit it's hard to adjust to going out in public and being triggered at first, but, when you're bringing along friends and having fun, you may just forget that you're in a "high risk" environment.

Mental Health

So many of our emotions are tied to our state of mental health. A good mood can help you to push triggers aside. If you're happy, you're less likely to let a trigger bring you into a state of depression or heightened anxiety. Mental health can bring a trigger from feeling like the apocalypse to feeling like a bump on the knee. This is one way that a therapist can be beneficial. They may not understand Misophonia, but they do understand how to help others to live a stress free life, and to make meaningful changes in order to feel happier, and more fulfilled, despite any challenges. The following are some ways in which your mental health can be helped:

Tips for Mental Health

» Drink tea. Whether it's red, green, or white, tea has been proven to have great benefits. It can significantly help stress, and even help your digestion. This is also a great way to reach your daily intake of water. If you believe that caffeine has a negative impact on your Misophonia, try herbal, caffeine free teas.

» Do yoga, or some other form of stress management. Yoga, Pilates, and other activities are great for your mind and your body.

» Find things you love. When you're doing things you love, the bad doesn't seem as bad. Even if there are triggers momentarily, you are much more likely to recover in an environment that makes you happy.

» Be creative. Creativity is like a cheap drug. You can paint, do crafts, photography, design, and just about anything that lets your brain wander and find interesting ideas to incorporate into an artistic form.

» Make goals and work toward them. When you're achieving life goals you will feel better about yourself. Especially when these goals are being met to spite your Misophonia. It can be a small goal, such as a healthier lifestyle, seeing your mother more, or a goal as large as starting your own business. The point is that working toward your goal will be good for your mind, and can help improve your life.

White Noise: This is used in some of the existing 'treatments' (there is no official cure or treatment, only experimental procedures). White noise is very important for eliminating audial triggers from an environment. Times like sleeping, being on a bus, or simply in day-to-day life can benefit from the addition of white noise. White noise can be found in the form of noise apps for phones, videos on a computer, fans, and white noise generators. Similarly, a TV or music may do the trick if you're merely trying to tune out trigger noises and cover them. There are also comforting sounds like ocean music and other 'calming' sounds. White noise may be more effective because it tends to block out our ability to hear these noises altogether, but music or a TV show can be helpful by creative a positive mood. It really depends on what you're looking for. Regardless of the noise that you choose to go with it is very useful to prevent hearing a trigger. White noise is most effective as a preventative measure, but can help lessen the effects once already triggered. Avoiding trigger sounds altogether is the best outcome, but that's not always possible. Remember that white noise will not take away the anger and discomfort that you are feeling toward a trigger, but it will help you from hearing more of the sound.

Distraction

This can be highly beneficial when trapped with a trigger. When you're in a car, on a bus, in class, or somewhere that you can't immediately leave, it's important to train your mind to focus on something else. It will not alleviate the entire trigger, but it can take your reaction from a ten to a two, if you're good at distracting yourself. You can distract yourself in many ways. Distraction is an important tool when you cannot get out of the situation. I have been known to put up my school bag as a barrier in classes, in order to avoid movements, and I am also known for wearing earplugs in classes, or playing games on my computer or chatting up a friend on my computer when I am trying to get away from the trigger environment mentally. A friend can help via text or a chat service, and you can really alter your mindset by making the time go by faster. This will not completely alleviate the trigger but it may make it a lot easier to deal with.

Support Groups

Support groups are a very tricky way to live with Misophonia. Acceptance from your peers is very important in learning to live with this condition, but the support groups also have negative effects that must be considered. It's very nice to know that you're not alone in your suffering. At first, these support groups will feel like a sanctuary. On a good day, they are filled with people giving helpful advice, kind phrases, and a loving attitude. On a bad day, they are vile pools of angry, distraught individuals fighting, and comments that attack one or more posters. Several persons with Misophonia use these support groups as a place to vent, while others merely want to experience a feeling of community. These ideals can clash. Support groups do have their place, but you must understand what you're getting into. Some of the larger groups have little to no moderation and have a greater chance of things turning sour, and fast. However, I run a support group entitled "Positive Misophonia Support". The goal here is to take out a lot of the bickering and have rules provided. There have been stories of people developing more triggers simply from reading the triggers of others.

Some groups feel the need to always alert you of a "trigger warning". This may be entirely counterproductive. Reading that there may be a trigger is very likely to engage your reflexes. You expect something bad to happen so you may very well be triggered no matter if it was initially a trigger. It is more appropriate to learn how to regulate your own sensory system instead of trying to police every aspect of your life.

Sometimes it is entirely legitimate to ask a person to stop something - such as the distracting behaviour of beating their fingers on a desk while you study. But, you musn't get trapped in the behaviour of avoiding triggers before they happen - this will lead you to the life of a hermit.

Coping Tips

Since there is no cure for Misophonia it is important that those who are sensory over-responsive (or under) are aware of their bodies. More evidence and research will need to be developed to ensure that a sensory diet can truly help Misophonia. However, in the mean time, it is a reasonable place to start. Many of the suggestions for a sensory diet can be helpful in other ways - reduced stress, reduced depression, and over-all heighened quality of life. The best part is - whether it works or not, there is little to no risk. It is just activities.

DO NOT try exposure therapy. There is a lot of evidence that Misophonia can be worsened by heightened exposure, and this seems to do little more than torture the patient.

Limit or avoid caffeine. Caffeine has been said to increase the feelings of Misophonia. Be mindful of caffeine and especially caffeine that has been combined with sugar or artificial sweeteners. Bring a music player, or have music on your phone, wherever you go. Try to find headphones that block out as much music as possible. When shopping, or on public transit, this can be very helpful.

Bring earplugs with you. I always have a pair in my pencil case, one in my purse, and another in my backpack. You never know when a moment may arise that is better with earplugs. I even use them in class. They block out most distracting noises, and if you're close enough to a speaker you can still hear them.

Snap a rubber band on your wrist. This is something that's

done for people with heightened anxiety, or who have problems with self- harm. Since Misophonia can have violent tendencies, this can be a form of release. However, if you have heightened violent feelings toward yourself or others, especially on a regular basis, please see a medical professional.

Put a physical blocker between you and the trigger. This is especially important for a visual trigger. Sometimes I'd have my friends move to block it, or I'd put up my hand. In classes I always sit with my backpack on the seat next to me, physically blocking the sight of triggers. This does not completely alleviate the feelings of anxiousness, but it has helped me to get through it.

Misophonia is a life-altering condition with no cure, therefore it's important that sufferers focus on what this means for them. It is important not to push these feelings away and feel guilty for having them. Grief must be dealt with, and allowed to go through its stages. Once you grieve, you can accept that this is not the end of the world and that you can still make a life for yourself. Grieving is not about giving up, it is about letting go, and moving forward with the changes that have to be made. There are five stages of grief that were originally proposed in the book On Death and Dying, in 1969, by Elisabeth Kübler-Ross. The stages of grief do not necessarily happen in order, and you can go from depression, back to anger, or any other combination.

The 5 Stages of Grief

1. Denial and Isolation: Denial can come in different ways.People with Misophonia may at first believe that they're just 'hyper- sensitive' or that it's their fault. Isolation is huge for Misophonia. A large number of sufferers spend most of their time alone, and choose jobs and activities where triggers will not bother them. While this may help to prevent triggers, it is not a meaningful way to spend all of your time. Personal relationships and social interactions are a large part of happiness. Alone time is great, but it should not be all of your time.

2. Anger: It makes sense to be angry with Misophonia. It's a life- changing, existence-altering condition. Even when you finally find out that you're not crazy and there's a name for it, you're faced with a harsh reality. There's currently no cure, and that's enough to make anybody angry. Of course it's not fair that you have to suffer from this, and that you can't just be 'normal'. However, the fact is, you have it, and you're going to have to move on. Yes, your anger is warranted. However, you can't risk the rest of your life and your happiness because of this condition.

3. Bargaining: Sufferers may try to find help in ways that have a small chance of working. This can involve using therapies that have either not been tested or approved, or have little evidence to support that they will work. This does not involve a logical process of trying to find help. While these methods can

be very helpful for personal acceptance, it is not helpful if done out of desperation. Lack of results may put you further down a path of anxiety and depression, and head your progress.

4. Depression: It's easy to get depressed when things seem so

bleak. Misophonia has been known to cause depression so severe that hopelessness and thoughts of suicide are possible. If this happens to you, you should contact a mental health professional. It is important that you are properly equipped with coping mechanisms to help you through these emotions. Depression from grief is normal, but if it becomes too intense and endangers your life, medical attention is a necessity. Do not feel guilty or be afraid that you might be judged if you need to ask for help. It shows great strength to seek the help that you need. Whether it is through therapy, or through soul searching, you must process your negative emotions and come to terms with them.

5. Acceptance: After you have gone through all of the stages of grief, it is important that you come to a realization. There's nothing you can do to change things. It's all right. Misophonia may be a chronic condition but that does not mean that you will not be able to live a meaningful life. Once you accept Misophonia it will be easier to focus on coping methods and creating the kind of life that you want to live.

Misophonia-Friendly Activities:

Living with Misophonia doesn't have to be a trap. You can live a full and happy life while dealing with this disorder. The following are activities that can be enjoyed, especially in environments where triggers may be minimal.

Bowling: If you're okay with the sound of the balls rolling and the pins crashing then bowling should be a good place to hang out with your friends. For those with visual triggers, it is usually dark during the evening bowling nights, especially on 'neon' or 'blacklight' nights that often happen on weekends. A bonus is that music and the sound of the crashing will most likely block out any small trigger noises.

Swimming: It's exercise, and it's fun. Swimming can be a great activity for those with Misophonia. However, you may not want to swim in a pool that is mostly filled with children if you do not like screaming. Also, some pools have lifeguards that are trigger happy with their whistles. Find a pool or a public beach that has minimum or no triggers and you should be able to enjoy a meaningful experience with your friends.

Staying In: Staying in with your friends doesn't have to be a boring experience. You can play video games, play board games, watch movies, cook together, have a mini party, and do whatever you enjoy at home, but with friends. This environment can be trigger free if you pre- warn your friends and ask them to respect your boundaries.

Nature Hike: If you're in an unpopulated area you can

enjoy nature with your friends, and let the scenery sink in. A possible trigger may be the sound of the birds, but if that doesn't bother you then you should be fine. Make sure that your companions are aware of your Misophonia and are willing to abstain from behaviors that may bother you

Malls: Hit or miss, depending on the nature of your triggers. But, I love malls because I can easily get out of a situation if it triggers me. There are so many sections and stores that I'm never forced to be with the same people for very long. It's easy to go to another store and forget about what happened. However, some people find stores and malls very irritating.

Places With High Trigger Levels

Unfortunately, not all places are Misophonia friendly. These places will not trigger every one but can be devastating for those that it does trigger. While now and then may be okay, some of these places should be avoided altogether if you are in a particularily heightened state beforehand. If the things that go on in these places heavily trigger you, you should not try to force it. Sometimes we have no choice but to go to a place that will trigger us. Below each section, there will be some tips for handling the situation if you find yourself forced to endure it, or if it is something you enjoy.

You need to find your personal limits. Do not force yourself to stay home merely because there "may be" a trigger. After-all, the world is an entirely huge place with lots of possibility. You may very well get hit by a car when crossing the street. Should you only ever go to stores on the right? Of course not. Risk is a part of life. Evaluate the risk of a situation based on your current mood and feelings. If you're having trouble seeing, due to fogged glasses, you may not want to cross the road until a) you can get your glasses cleaned or b) another day when it is not foggy, since you do not need what is on the otehr side very much. However, if you truly need something on the other side of the road, you may decide to "suck it up". Misophonia requires checking in with yourself.

Theatres: Chewing, shuffling feet, people's silhouette's moving in the dark, and maybe some seat kicking. Depending on your triggers, the theatre can be a nightmare. However, some people find going to theatres can be manageable with the headphones that are used for disabilities. You can contact your local theatre to ask if they offer them before going.

If you do go there:

Try to get the headphones for sound

Sit near the back so that you do not have people behind you Try to be near friends so you will not feel alone

Restaurants: Unfortunately, restaurants are breeding grounds for triggers. Both visual and audial triggers are in abundance at most restaurants. If you're lucky, you can find a nice booth in a quiet back corner, but if you're going during regular business hours, you may be in for an unpleasant experience. The only pleasant dining experiences I have had in restaurants in the past 2 years have been at odd hours, and when I happened to be the only patron. I recommend take-out, pick-up, or delivery if you really want to splurge on restaurant food.

If you do go there:

Try to sit away from the kitchen, there is a lot of noise from these workers

Try to sit at the back of a booth, with your friends on the outside to act as a buffer for triggers

Get a table in a corner away from others

Try to go at times when there are usually less diners, such as 3pm

Waiting Rooms: These places are full of triggers. People in waiting rooms tend to be anxious and their nervous ticks can become full-blown triggers for a person with Misophonia. I try to avoid waiting rooms as best as possible. Waiting rooms are an unfortunate fact of life, and should be avoided if they can. However, if you need to be in a waiting room, chances are you have to go there. If it is for a government document or paper, first check to see if you can get this service done via mail.

If you do go there:

Sit in the back, or in a corner

If you can, have a friend sit next to you in order to block out other people

Try to book appointments in the early morning or mid afternoon. These times people are usually at work, and not at appointments

Public Transportation: Hot, stuffy, and cramped with people. Public transportation whether trains, busses, or planes, is filled with Misophonia triggers. Those of us who have no other choice are forced into this awful situation, sometimes multiple times a day.

If you do go there:

Try to go when there is less people, if not possible, try to sit as far away from people as possible and isolate yourself. I usually use my backpack on my lap and look out the window

Sit in the back, or in a corner

If you can, have a friend sit next to you in order to block out other people

DISCLAIMER

Since there is no official cure, there may be people who claim that he or she can help sufferers to alleviate all of their symptoms. To a person who has been suffering all their life, these cures can sound like a miracle and mimic the trend of the dieting industry. These people are looking for your money, and they are not to be trusted. This does not mean that all "cures" are scams or fake, but it does mean that you have to be weary.

If a person approaches you offering a cure, you should not accept just because it seems like a miracle cure. Actually, you should be quite disgruntled, as "miracle cures" do not exist for this condition. Most doctors do not approach patients; even researchers are unlikely to do so because they understand the ethics involved with offering experimental treatments. Unfortunately, a doctorate or medical practice does not mean that the person has significant working knowledge of Misophonia.

Awareness

Action is the foundational key to all success. - Picasso

Since Misophonia is only a newly recognized condition, it is important that the doctors who study it, and the people who suffer from it, are advocating for awareness. Some believe that awareness will lead to negative individuals acting inappropriately against sufferers, but with proper advocacy, this should be alleviated.

Awareness is important for all disorders and conditions. This is evident in the growing support for mental illness, and the need for open dialogue and understanding. Of course the entire world will never be able to change in order to help those who have Misophonia, but through awareness we will further incentives for research and for plans that can genuinely help those with Misophonia.

In my own experience, Misophonia has been much easier to manage now that I can tell family and friends what is wrong. Like a good diet, healthy and understanding friends and family can lead to an overall improvement in quality of life. It's important that the people you interact with know that there is currently no cure. Therapy might help, but it will not eliminate symptoms.

Once upon a time, many of the disorders we are now aware of and actively work to alleviate today were considered abnormal and strange. Misophonia may currently be considered abnormal or strange, but as awareness grows, it may become a stigma of the past. There may be initial downfall at first. The more awareness that grows, it may at first be considered odd and a piece of gossip. All things must go through this phase. In order to have gains we must be prepared for the potential losses.

Awareness isn't some magical concept that can be achieved simply by wanting it to happen. If we want Misophonia to be a widely understood and accepted condition, we must be willing to talk about it. Like all illnesses that have been stigmatized, it starts with a conversation.

It can be difficult to talk about Misophonia. There's a lot of pressure when you know that the person on the receiving end probably won't understand what you're going through. That doesn't mean you shouldn't try. Everyone can help raise awareness for Misophonia. It starts with your family and friends, your community, your school or workplace. At first, it may be seen as a strange word, a strange disorder, or an annoyance. Over time, it will grow to be something familiar. Information and exposure are the only way that a person's mind can be changed. Of course, there'll always be the naysayers, the doubters and the people who refuse to respect your illness – but these people exist in all lifestyles, for all reasons. There was once a time when it was okay to label a disabled person as retarded. Now, that's so unspeakable that I considered using asterisks for some of the letters. There was also a time when people with depression and anxiety were told to suck it up, and there was a time just few decades ago where these people may have spent their lives in an asylum. The world is changing, but it isn't changing through suffering in silence.

It is my belief that access to information is an important way to spread the word about this illness. Posts that can be shared, posts about information, and graphic images are used to help those who suffer from Misophonia share information with their friends and families. For me, what's most important is that people know that this is more than a condition and a label; Misophonia is a life-altering disorder that can seriously impede quality of life. This book was written for the purpose of awareness. It is through information that we will change how the world views this disorder.

In Beyond The Label, stigma is discussed in detail. Stigma is more than just how a person feels about a disorder, it has a great impact on the life of the sufferer. While Misophonia is not the same as mental illness, there is little else to compare it to – and since the reactions appear mental (to an onlooker), it can be put under the same umbrella as many mental illnesses. Below is the definition of stigma in a book designated for raising awareness and cutting away the label for mental illness and addiction.

Stigma is not merely a problem of "hurting people's feelings." Stigma interferes with the person's full participation in society, can lead to and/or increase mental health and substance use problems, and can provoke the person to withdraw from relationships and services that could be helpful. Stigma can seriously hamper matters such as holding a job, having a home, accessing services and participating in social relationships (CAMH)

The fear of being judged and scrutinized can stop people from looking for help. Since Misophonia is not a well known condition, it can be very isolating attempting to search for a cure, and even worse, when they find out there is not one. This is why awareness is so important – awareness can remove stigma, both from the medical community and from the public. Without research, Misophonia will remain a relatively unknown condition, and without advocacy, the demand for research is lowered. The more doctors, graduate students, and people that have heard of

Misophonia, the greater chance of finding a cure, or helping sufferers to handle the disorder properly.

Here are some ways that you can help raise awareness for Misophonia. On the Misophonia Awareness site, we will be posting new ways for people to get involved. However, you don't have to wait to start making a difference.

Social Media

You may think that social media's best attributes are sharing game invites to friends, and connecting with your long-lost childhood friend. That may be true, but it also has a plethora of resources for raising awareness. The ability to post, like, and share has allowed many organizations to get their messages across. The more people that hear about Misophonia, the greater chance that doctors and researchers will learn about it.

Social media is an amazingly powerful platform. Anybody, anywhere, at any time, can connect and share a vision and an idea. It is easy to spread awareness and content with people whom you may never have met without social media. Through Twitter, Google +, and Facebook you can reach a wider audience and ensure that the message of Misophonia gets out there. I recommend that you follow the Misophonia Awareness page on these sites and share our content with your friends and families.

Your Community

You may be surprised to learn that your own community holds opportunities to raise awareness. You can ask to set up an information booth at several functions, whether they are BBQs, advocacy events, or merely community parties. You can raise a lot of awareness by having pamphlets, posters, and other items to promote awareness. Support materials will be available through MisophoniaAwareness.org.

Friends and Family

Your friends and family can provide a great backdrop for explaining your disorder. Remember that each person you tell will be able to tell another, and then another. Simply explaining Misophonia to others can be both cathartic and a way to spread awareness.

Your School/Workplace

Like the sources mentioned above, you may be surprised at the awareness you can spread just by talking to your work-mates/classmates, and other professionals. These people may also have great resources that you can take advantage of. This provides a wonderful opportunity for networking. Besides, you never know what somebody will be working on down the road, and how you can be mutually beneficial.

They are:

Respect the person as an individual. Chances are they are not trying to trigger you, and merely have little to no under-standing of the disorder.

Try not to approach a person who is triggering you with a discussion on Misophonia when you are triggered. If you must say something, take a breath and remain calm. Politely ask the person to stop. Do not verbally attack the person.

Understand why the person makes the noise and do not disregard their feelings. Say you understand, but that it is a medical condition and that you would really appreciate if they would be willing to help you.

Do not apologize for your disorder. This takes away cred-ibility and makes it seem like there is something you can do differently.

Explaining Misophonia

Since Misophonia isn't a widely known disorder, it is important that those who suffer are well equipped to explain their condition to parties who could be causing a trigger, or to those who are able to provide support for Misophonia. This chapter will aim to provide suggestions for explaining the condition to different parties, and will suggest ways to avoid a negative situation. It is important that you feel respected by every one that you interact with. Of course, this can be difficult when dealing with strangers – but when it comes to people, you have a personal or professional relationship with, respect must be maintained.

Tips for all people you have to deal with, regardless of who assertive when you state that you have a neurological condition. You can be polite and assertive at the same time.

Explain that Misophonia does not mean that you are making excuses for yourself, it merely means that you are taking your health into your own hands.

If a person does not understand but shows interest, offer to send them links to sites on Misophonia (you can find these in the 'resources' chapter of the book). Tell them that it's reasonable that they don't know, but that there is growing research on the disorder. Before arranging to meet with a new person I briefly explain my disorder. I explain that certain sights and sounds give me a fight or flight reaction, and ask that they keep them to a minimum. I have had much more ease explaining this before meeting, than in the moment when being triggered, which is essentially too late.

Friends

I now refuse to spend time recreationally with people who do not respect my Misophonia. It was a hard adjustment at first – but the people who truly care about me are able to respect my condition. Friendship, like dating, should be based on a mutual understanding and trust. You should not have to pressure your friend to respect your needs and wishes, and your friend should not feel attacked by your sudden rage at noises or visuals. Be sure to explain to your friend that you do not mean anything by your displeasure, and that you truly value their time and your relationship. Ask if you can have gatherings in trigger-neutral zones, and plan your outings so that the possibility of a trigger is minimal. This can be hard, since a lot of friendships involve activities that involve noises or visual stimuli. Try to pick outings that have noises that you are comfortable with. For example, I'm fine with the sound of bowling balls and pins crashing. Bowling is a great way to hang out with friends because most of the people I can see are standing – which means not shaking any body parts, and the rest of the facility is usually dark. A great friend will understand that you are not doing this to be nitpicky and will want to make you feel better. However, you must understand that they have emotions too, and that you should try not to attack them when triggered.

Romantic Partner

Ah, romance, the place where we're supposed to accept the other individual regardless of their inconsistent behaviors. Misophonia is the devil in your ear nagging at you. Your partner clinks their spoon in a bowl, taps their fingers, or shakes their leg. Maybe they like to whistle. At first, you may try to ignore it, but eventually the triggers can become worse and worse. The honeymoon is over, and Misophonia changes all of your emotions. Like friends and family, you need to be able to discuss your Misophonia with your partner. Hard work and honesty are going to be the key in going forward. Your partner must respect your condition and how the role it plays in your life, and you must understand and respect your partner's emotions when it comes to being the trigger, and living their life with you.

Family

Those nearest and dearest are often the worst triggers. We spend a lot of time with our loved ones, and in general, we seem less forgiving when it comes to their behaviours. Day in and day out with the same people can be stressful for any situation. Even if you do not live with a family member, the intensity of the relationship can still cause Misophonia triggers to be worse. My first ever "trigger person" that I knew of was my mother. At first, every time she shook her foot, it was a major fight. We're talking volcanic eruption on both sides. You didn't want to be there when she played music and when she sang. I know it isn't her fault that she does these things, and they never used to bother me. Misophonia doesn't always make sense.

Roommates

Like family, these people are there on a day-to-day basis. However, unlike family, there may not be enough of a personal relationship that you can confront the individual in a positive manner. Sometimes our living arrangements are out of our control. You may be living in a dorm room, an apartment, or another communal situation. Money, and other uncontrollable forces often lead to the necessity of living with a stranger, or even an acquaintance. Ideally, we would never live with someone whom we didn't have a good relationship with. Unfortunately, reality isn't always a perfect picture. If you're going to be living with a new person, you should discuss your Misophonia before moving in. Try to be sure that the person you're going to live with truly understands your needs, and establish ground rules. Explain that you are not trying to dictate them and that you are merely suffering from a neurological condition. If they, or a current roommate, do not respect these ground rules, perhaps you should consider a different living arrangement, if possible. Living with your triggers should be only a last resort. While you cannot avoid triggers in every aspect of your life, the home should be a neutral place where you can relax and have a sanctuary, for the sake of your health and sanity.

Boss or Administration

Your boss should be a person that you trust and that you can approach with issues that involve your work performance and comfort in the workplace. For some people, their boss is intimidating and a person that they would rather not confront. Either way, it is best to go into this conversation prepared. You should explain Misophonia is a neurological condition that can't be helped, though there is little information and no cure yet. Ask your boss if there is anything they can do to help, and assure them that, you are committed to the job, and are asking for the betterment of not just you, but your performance. If your boss is not supportive, you should be armed on the laws reflecting accessibility in your region.

Co-Workers

Co-workers can be tricky. You have to play nice when you have a job. This is especially worrisome for those that work in an office environment. A lot of workplaces are starting to allow snacking on the job, and this causes a lot of triggers. Being polite can go a long way with other workers, no matter the situation. However, sometimes coworkers aren't willing to stop something that they believe is 'their right'. Approach the coworker when you aren't triggered and inform them that you have a medical condition, and ask them if they would be willing to help accommodate you. If they are not willing to help and further the situation, inform your boss. You should already have told your boss about your Misophonia and discussed the possibility of accommodations. If you are lucky, you may be able to convince your boss to speak with your co-worker. Remind everyone involved Misophonia a neurological condition that you cannot control.

Doctors (and other Medical Professionals)

When faced with a medical struggle, most of us decide to go to a doctor. The trouble with Misophonia is that many doctors have never heard of it. Most doctors will automatically assume that it is psychological and will refer you to a psychiatrist or a psychologist, or personally recommend a medication. This can be frustrating, and possibly infuriating. Depending on where you live, it may cost a lot of money to be thrown through hoops without knowing if you'll ever find a cure. It's best to do your research on doctors that provide help for Misophonia. However, you should still have a conversation with your doctor and let them know what is happening with you. As research grows, your doctor may become interested in the illness, and could eventually help others, and maybe even you.

Teachers and Professors

For those of you lucky enough to be out of the school game, I salute you. Dealing with professors and teachers can be its own kind of hell. Thankfully, most schools these days (at least Universities, Colleges, and Technical Schools), have great accessibility programs. They're not perfect, but they're getting a lot better. The hardest part of this seems to be intimidation. The entire system seems set up to make professors and teachers seem larger than life, and that can be intimidating. If your school wants you to discuss your condition with your professor, you must approach them when you are in a good mood. You should never approach your professor on a day in which you are triggered. I have been lucky enough to only have positive interactions with my professors in regards to my Misophonia, anxiety, and depression. Remember that most teachers and professors are there to help you. They are not the enemy, and they want their students to succeed. All of your interactions should be polite, considerate, and professional. Speak to the professor with kindness but with firmness.

Going Into The Conversation

When you know that you have to tell a person about your disorder, it can be stressful – the anxiety, fear, and anticipation can be enough to keep your mouth firmly shut, and continue your suffering. However, it's important that you go through with it. Keeping things bottled up will not help your disorder, or your life – I promise you that. Consider the tips below when you're going to confront somebody. You may want to adjust the conversation depending on whom you're talking to, but these tips should help you when thinking about how to act, what to do, and what to say. It's a good idea to make sure you're not triggered at the time of the conversation. During a trigger, your anger is heightened and you may perceive the person as a threat. It's important that you are prepared to explain Misophonia in a positive manner. No one wants to feel attacked.

Prepare yourself with research and website links that can be helpful to explain Misophonia to the person you're about to approach. Make sure that they will understand that it is a real condition, and that you are serious.

Keep your mood stress-free, and ensure that you are relaxed beforehand. Try to have a bath, some tea, and some light television or something you enjoy before you have the conversation. If you're stressed or tired, the conversation may go south quickly. It is important that you are in a good mood for the conversation. Choose a location in which you know there will be little to no triggers. Try to be somewhere that you and the other individual are both comfortable. If this is not possible, try to become familiar with the place beforehand (such as talking to the person in their office before-hand, and asking if you can meet another day, when you have more time, or are prepared).

During The Conversation

During the conversation, your aim should be to keep it positive and informative. You should provide examples of what trigger you, even if they are not the same ones that trigger you in the environment with the person. It's important that they understand it is not just when you are around this person, and that this disorder impacts several aspects of your life. Do not make it all about them.

It may be helpful to print off articles that explain Misophonia, and what it is. Since research is minimum, some of the websites listed at the end of this book can be helpful for learning about Misophonia. If the person triggers you during the conversation, identify it but not in an aggressive manner. Excuse yourself, and explain that what they are doing is one of the things that cause a reaction. Politely ask if they can stop or if there is a way, they can adjust their behaviour. Make sure they understand you are not blaming them, but that the condition is serious.

Do not apologize for Misophonia or make excuses. Say that it is a neurological condition, and that you have it. Be matter-of-fact, and explain that unfortunately there is no cure.

Discuss a way that you can let them know you are being triggered, without being offensive, or turning to anger.

If the conversation starts to go sour, or the person does not understand – excuse yourself. Do not let anger turn into a confrontation. Explain that you were merely explaining your feelings, and that this has a huge impact on your life. Leave before it becomes more serious, often leaving is a statement of its own.

After the Conversation

Chances are, after you explain Misophonia to another person, they will still trigger you. It can be hard for a person to recondition things that they are used to doing, and even harder to remember. Unlike you, this person does not deal with Misophonia on a day-in-day-out basis, so it's unlikely that it's something they consider regularly. Do not blame them for this, and do not hold it against them. Unless the person is trying to trigger you and disregards your feelings entirely, you should be mindful that they are probably not out to get you, and that is merely a reaction from Misophonia.

» If you have to remind them that they are triggering you, be polite.

» Leave the room and if they ask why, explain that you're being triggered.

» Try to remain positive; do not engage when you are angry.

The Other Side Of The Fence

I get it, explaining Misophonia to another person is a hard thing to do. It can send us into a panic. We don't want to be judged, and we're worried about the reaction of the person we're confronting. But, have you considered what the reaction of the other person may be, and why? I know you're worried that it will be a lack of understanding and negative – but why would it be negative? Hearing a sufferer explain her condition, but also, how she changes her lifestyle for her son gave me some ideas. For once, I wasn't the person explaining that I had the disorder; I was merely the person listening to the story. As well, I've read all the interviews in this book and had conversations with a lot of sufferers. To say the least, it was strange to be on the other side of the fence. This is the side where you don't exactly know what to say, and you're at a loss for word. In this section, I want to shed some light on this position. Hopefully, I can also help people without the disorder to understand what they could say to get around their confusion. There's a good chance that the person who is triggering you does not want you to feel such a negative reaction from their behaviour. Even worse, they may feel guilty, or like they're being blamed for your thoughts and feelings, and that can be troublesome to live with. The following are considerations to make about the feelings of people who are your triggers, and what it may be like to be them.

I haven't always had Misophonia. I can still remember the days of old when I wasn't bothered by or triggered by any noises. A person who doesn't have sensory processing issues or Misophonia probably won't notice the sights or sounds that you're noticing. In fact, they may be so oblivious that they don't even know if they're making noise or moving. When you have Misophonia it's nearly impossible to imagine that these noises or visuals can be completely unseen and unheard. However, when you're not living with it on a daily basis, it can be very hard to understand what the big deal is about. A person without Misophonia may wonder why you're so upset and first think you're merely hypersensitive. It's not their fault that they think this way. Each person has trouble seeing outside of his or her own experiences, so it's hard to consider the viewpoint of a person with Misophonia.

A person who is triggering a loved one or a close friend may feel a significant amount of guilt when trying to deal with Misophonia and its impact on their loved one. After all, they do not want to hurt you, and yet, one wrong move and they're being given the stink-eye, again. It's traumatic to always be griped at and 'attacked' for making a noise you're used to, or moving a body part. Unfortunately, the person who is triggered has little control of their rage in the moment. However, that doesn't mean that the feelings of the person who the rage is directed toward do not feel it too. People have trouble considering changing their habits or behaviours in order to ease the lifestyle of another. It's not because they're arrogant or selfish, it's because everybody is just trying to get by, in their own way. A significant amount of the population hums, whistles, or shakes their legs or sways when they are uncomfortable or faced with anxiety. Unfortunately, these behaviours tend to send people with Misophonia into a rage, and this reaction could further send the person causing the trigger into anxiety. Misophonia is uncomfortable for everybody involved.

The lack of medical knowledge and research on Misophonia is not only challenging, but also very confusing for people who do no have it. If you think it's hard living with the disorder, imagine watching it happen but not knowing what to do, or whether or not your actions could actually be making the disorder worse. This is especially challenging for parents that are trying to guide their children in the right direction. A lot of people will say that their kids cannot be coddled and that they should be forcing them to 'toughen up'. This can send a mixed message to parents. Since the pain associated with Misophonia is severe, a parent's reaction will be to protect their child – but a lot of people will be urging them to force their child to 'get over it'. All current findings on Misophonia believe that the disorder gets worse with exposure. It'll be impossible to keep a child away from any and all triggers, but forcing them to deal with it is not the way to go. There's a fine line between avoiding life and purposefully exposing a person to triggers. Balance should be found that helps each person, and there is no "one-size-fits-all" to take care of Misophonia.

Misophonia is an emotional struggle for everybody involved. There are no right answers, and the current amount of research and diagnosis is so small that it's hard to feel a sense of hope once you know that it's in-fact a real diagnosis. However, this does not mean that everything has to be gray skies. Open communication can be helpful for everybody. If you are being triggered, you should be able to communicate positively and if it's the only excuse, leave the room. If you are not the person suffering, but rather the trigger, or a person involved with a Misophonia sufferer, you should learn not to take their behaviour personally.

Here are some things to think about, in regards to Misophonia. This is broken into two sections. The first is for loved ones, and the second is for sufferers. I recommend you each read both so that you can get a full picture of the situation. Understanding is an important way to have a harmonious relationship.

For Loved Ones

If you are triggering your loved one, do not treat them as though it is simply his or her problem and that they have to get over it. Acknowledge that it is a real problem, and if you are unable to adjust what you are doing, at least be mindful of their emotions.

If your loved one leaves the room, or excuses his or herself from an event or a conversation, either momentarily or for long periods of time, try not to make them feel guilty. Misophonia is very sensitive to exposure and it should be encouraged that the person feels safe and comfortable in finding the right balance for his or her life. It is important that a person with Misophonia knows that they are able to escape, and that they are not trapped or isolated in the situation.

Try not to feel guilty. It is not your fault that your loved one has this disorder. However, it may be your actions causing the trigger, it is not your fault that it is happening, it is Misophonia that causes this reaction, and you have nothing to feel guilty for.

If you are having difficulty explaining Misophonia to other family members or friends who do not understand the reaction of your loved one, explain to them that it is a neurological condition and that your loved ones brain simply interprets certain noises and sounds differently than others, and that they see them as a threat. Explain that this reaction is usually both physical as well as emotional, that the rage is felt immediately, and that they are unable to control it.

Consider family counseling. Although a counselor will not be able to cure Misophonia, they may be able to help your family develop ways of understanding each other. Misophonia tends to lead to a self-centered attitude in sufferers, due to the nature of the disorder. It can be helpful to have a therapist that understands at least some sensory processing issues. It is important that you, and your entire family, know how to communicate and express emotions in a positive and mindful manner.

If it's been a heated day for you and the sufferer, consider taking a mini-vacation from them. It may be watching a movie in another room or removing you or the sufferer from the environment. While you're apart, it can be nice if you're both doing something you love and enjoy. When you come back together you may both be ready to talk in a pleasurable manner, or at least, without taking each other's throats out.

For Sufferers

You must remember that your loved one has emotions too. Yes, you are angry and triggered by an action. However, your loved one is impacted by this disorder as well. Significant life changes happen on either side, and it is important that you are mindful of theirsacrifices and the negativity that they must deal with. Even though it is not your fault that you feel this way you cannot discount the other person's feelings.

You shouldn't feel guilty for leaving a family event, or a friend's house. If you have to get out of a situation, that's that. Unlike anxiety, it will not help you to push through a trigger. However, if a trigger is not going to last long, like fireworks, brief scene on TV or other momentary things, it is reasonable to stay. However, if you are being consistently triggered and feel your mood getting worse and worse, and the angry heightening, it is wise to get to safer pastures and wait out the storm.

If your Misophonia is causing a rift in a relationship, try not to feel guilty. While you cannot change how you act in a trigger situation, or at least not a lot, you can change how you behave after the situation. Be mindful of the emotions of the other person and be sure that you're willing to negotiate parameters and ground rules for how you deal with the situation. Having a plan can help everybody involved know what's going to go down, and there will be fewer hard feelings later. Any bumps that happen can be discussed, instead of fought over.

Like mentioned for the loved ones, family counseling can

be a great way to help everybody talk through their feelings and discuss their emotions in a positive and effective manner. If therapy is not available because of cost or other restraints, you can simply Google ways to discuss important family matters, or come up with a plan that works best for your family, and sit down and talk it out.

Another repeat from the above section: take a break from the person who is triggering you. Go to a friend's, go to your own room, or go for a walk outside. It's not helping anybody if you're staying in a negative situation.

Current Research

The Roots, Influences and Future Possibilities of Misophonia Research

By Dr. Jennifer Jo Brout

To date, Misophonia has mostly garnered attention from researchers in audiology, Obsessive Compulsive and Related Disorders, Anxiety, and Synesthesia. In audiology, research both addresses the similarities and distinctions between Hyperacusis and Misophonia. In psychology, commonalities between Obsessive Compulsive and Related Disorders and anxiety are currently being investigated. In neuroscience, models of Misophonia as a form of Synesthesia are proposed. Across this research is also discussion of "general sensory sensitivities," "sensory-defensiveness" and "multisensory processing" (e.g. Wu, Lewin, Murphy, & Storch, 2014). The research in Misophonia is in its infancy but can be grossly categorized into Audiology/Otology, Psychology, Psychiatry and Neuroscience. This is not a full literature review, but is instead a summary of relevant work.

The beginning of Misophonia Research

Problems with Terminology

The term Misophonia, which means "hatred of sound,"

was first coined by Jastreboff and Jastreboff (2001). Dr. Pawel Jastreboff is a Professor of Otology (Head and Neck Surgery) at Emory University, and Margaret Jastreboff holds a PhD in biology (and has post doctoral training in pharmacology and molecular biology). Yet, emphasis in new research focuses mostly on how they went about "terming the disorder" and not on their theory.

For example, M. Johnson, an Audiologist who practices in the U.S., feels that the disorder should be called Selective Sound Sensitivity Syndrome or "4S". Dr. Johnson has seen Misophonia patients for over ten years, has kept careful clinical notes and clearly has a point. Misophonia does not describe the disorder accurately (personal correspondence, 2015) as people with Misophonia do not hate "all sounds." Rather, they have highly aversive reactions to specific patterned-based sounds, and some are also over-responsive to visual stimuli. Notably, there is now a name for aversive responsivity to movement (as "seen" through the visual sense) called Misokinesia, termed by Arjan Schroder (2014). So, as is the case in the health, mental health, and all the allied fields, we struggle with continual changing definitions and terminology, complicating our ability to understand that which is incomprehensible, even to our greatest scientists.

Audiology/Otology

Research in this area is mainly confined to the Jastreboffs' work. However, it is very important to understand their theory, as it is both the catalyst for interest in Misophonia and has been subject to a great deal of misinterpretation. The Jastreboffs defined Misophonia while treating patients with tinnitus (ringing in the ears) and hyperacusis (severe intolerance for loud sounds). The Jastreboff's made a very important distinction, specifically between Hyperacusis and Misophonia. Hyperacusis patients aversely react to loud noises whereas Misophonics react to "repetitive or pattern based noises" regardless of decibel level (Jastreboff & Jastreboff, 2014). This is the first important distinction:

Misophonia – aversive response to repetitive and patterned based sounds that may often be quiet, or "soft."

Hyperacusis – aversive response to loud sounds.

According to the Jastreboff's both conditions are subsumed under "Decreased Sound Tolerance" and both conditions relate to "aberrant" or "atypical" associations between the auditory and the limbic system (the limbic system is known to be the "emotional center" of the brain). However, regarding Hyperacusis, the Jastreboff's hypothesized that the brain circuitry involved was purely subconscious. That is, the brain regions and connections amongst these brain structures/regions were completely out of control of the "conscious" or "thinking part" of our brain.

To simplify, in hyperacusis one part of the brain is telling the other to perceive sounds much more loudly than they really are, and this is going on without any involvement of the part of the brain that is involved in conscious thought (where more sophisticated kinds of memory and organization that only human beings are capable of occurs). The next important distinction made by the Jastreboffs':

Misophonia: Abnormal connections amongst auditory, emotional and part of brain (often referred to as the limbic system).

Hyperacusis – Abnormal connection in auditory and emotional part of the brain (often referred to as the "limbic system")

In addition, unlike hyperacusis patients who responded to loud noises all the time, Misophonics seem varied in their responses. That is, the patients the Jastreboffs treated reported a variety of emotions in response to sounds, ranging from annoyance to rage, and including fear and avoidance of situations/

places in which trigger sounds might be present, and numerous other mixed descriptors. The Jastreboff's also noted that their patients reacted to some people and not others (and in some places but not others). This led them to believe that Misophonic individuals had made negative associations between specific noises and specific people, or between specific noises and particular experiences and/or places. They theorized that this meant that these responses were "learned". This is where the more conscious part of the brain (or the "cortical structures") becomes relevant.

Simplified, in the Jastreboff's view sounds (processed in the "auditory part of the brain") were associated during a negative experience with a person, place or experience within the limbic system (the "emotional part of the brain) and then stored in memory (via the "cortical structures"). Once this negative association is formed, every time the same sound is encountered, a person with Misophonia will experience autonomic arousal. Autonomic arousal refers to physiological arousal associated with what is commonly referred to as the "fight or flight" syndrome (although it can be experienced at lower levels without fight/flight occurring).

The Jastreboffs' did not venture to study Misophonia "in a lab" in order to support their theory, but instead began treating patients under the assumption that although Misophonia is a neurologically based disorder, the negative associations that have been made between the sounds and the particular experiences could be re-trained through making new and positive associations with sounds.

Psychology/Psychiatry and Neuroscience

In psychology, Obsessive Compulsive and Related Disorders have also received attention in the small but growing body of literature on Misophonia. Schröder, Vulink, and Denys (2013) recruited 42 patients who self-reported Misophonia symptoms. They were interviewed by a psychiatrist and given various measures pertaining to neuropsychiatric diagnosis. Notably, the authors found the highest incidence of overlap with the DSM-IV TR Obsessive Compulsive Personality Disorders. Specifically, results from this study indicated the level of comorbidity with other psychiatric maladies. Out of 42 Dutch patients, 7.1% Mood disorders, 2.4% panic disorder, 4.8% ADHD, 2.4% OCD and 52.4% OCPD was reported (Schroder, 2013). Schröder et al. (2013) also found the following attributes in the group of 42 Misophonics: 1) aversive and angry feelings evoked by particular sounds, 2) rare potentially aggressive outbursts, 3) recognition by the Misophonic individual that his/her behavior is excessive, 4) avoidance behavior, and 5) distress and interference in daily life.

Schröder, et al. (2013) proposed that Misophonia should be considered a discrete disorder under the broader classification Obsessive and Compulsive Related Disorders in the DSM-5. The researchers were recruited from a mental health clinic, which may have biased their sample (Jastreboff & Jastreboff, 2014). In addition, it is too early in the stage of research to label Misophonia as a psychiatric disorder, and we must take into consideration new conceptualizations of dimensional versus categorical classification regarding mental health (Insel, 2012). Notably, the authors recognized a symptom overlap with SPD, but their quantitative analysis may have been impacted by a misunderstanding of SPD/SOR. Specifically, in their description of SPD they state that individuals with SPD only react to "loud" sounds and not to the repetitive sounds (the sounds indicated in Misophonia). This is not true. The research in SPD, specifically on SOR children, does not differentiate between loud or patterned noises. This is an issue that has not yet been parsed out in SPD/SOR research and therefore assumptions such as this should not be made.

Wu, Lewin, Murphy, and Storch (2014) investigated the incidence, phenomenology, correlates, and level of impairment associated with Misophonia symptoms in 483 undergraduate students through self-report measures. In their sample, nearly 20% of participants reported clinically significant Misophonic symptoms. These symptoms were strongly associated with measures of general life impairment and sensory sensitivities, as well as moderate associations with obsessive-compulsive, anxiety, and depressive symptoms. The authors report that the symptom association with sensory sensitivities may indicate that selective sound sensitivities may be linked to higher occurrences of other types of sensory defensiveness as well (Baguley & McFerran, 2011; Stansfeld, Clark, Jenkins & Tarnopolsky, 1985). In addition, the authors report that anxiety mediated the relationship between misophonia and anger outbursts. Finally, as limitations to their study, the authors note that most study participants were female and that only self-report measures were used.

Edelstein, Brang, Rouw, and Ramachandran (2013) found similarities between Synesthesia and Misophonia. Edelstein et al. proposed that Misophonia "displays similarities" to synesthesia. Edelstein et al. used both self-report (qualitative interviews) and physiologic measures (Skin Conductance Response, or SCR) to measure reactivity in Misophonia. "In synesthesia, as in Misophonia, particular sensory stimuli evoke particular and consistent, additional sensations and association. In short, a pathological distortion of connections between the auditory cortex and limbic structures could cause a form of sound-emotion synesthesia" (Edelstein et al., 2013).The authors note that limitations of the study include small sample size, a lack of screening for psychiatric or psychological problems (no measures of mental health disorders were included), and that SCR measures autonomic arousal, but does not describe the nature of the emotion associated with that autonomic arousal.

Sensory Processing Disorder and Misophonia: The Overlap

It is also important to note that there is a remarkable overlap in Misophonia symptoms and Sensory Over-Responsivity (SOR), a subtype of Sensory Processing Disorder (SPD). Work in SPD began in the field of Occupational Therapy but has expanded to include neuroscience, psychology, psychiatry, and genetics over the past 15 years. This impressive body of research supports that particular groups of young children misperceive auditory, visual, tactile and other stimuli as highly aversive and dangerous. Notably, the research in SOR has been related mainly to children, although currently it is beginning to address adults as well.

While SOR research concerns a variety of sensory stimuli, it is important to note that within these groups were children known as mainly "auditory over-responsive." There are numerous papers that focus on auditory over-responsive symptoms, as well as studies focused specifically on auditory gating (e.g. Gavin, W. J., Dotseth, A., Roush, K. K., Smith, C. A., Spain, H. D., & Davies, P. L., 2011). SPD/SOR research, even that which was specific to the auditory modality, did not differentiate between loud and repetitive sounds. This makes it difficult to extrapolate from SOR to Misophonia. However, the overlap in behavioral symptoms in regard to "auditory over-responsivity" is remarkable.

Brief History of SOR research

As far back as 1999 studies of children considered SOR demonstrated autonomic arousal and decreased habituation. Specifically, measured by electro dermal reactivity (EDR) children who presented with every day sensory stimuli and responses were measured by galvanic skin responses. Many children with SOR exhibited increased amplitude, frequency and reduced habituation to sensory stimulation (e.g. McIntosh, Miller, Shyu, & Hagerman, 1999; James, Miller, Schaff, Neilsen, & Schoen, 2011). Notably, these and other studies of SOR children have been replicated over the past 15 years, and have included numerous other physiologic and brain imaging studies showing differences between typicals and SOR children, as well differences between typical children and children with more general atypical sensory processing problems (e.g. Davies & Gavin, 2007; Davies et al., 2009, 2010; Davies, Chang, & Gavin, 2009; Gavin et al., 2011; Van Hulle, Schmidt, & Goldsmith, 2012; Owen et al., 2013; Schnieder et al., 2009).

Because SPD is not yet validated by psychiatry (e.g., is not included in the DSM-5), this impressive body of literature is often overlooked in psychiatric and psychology research. This is despite the past decades of SPD scholarship, which includes contributions from esteemed researchers within psychiatry, psychology, and basic science (e.g. Goldsmith et al., 2006, Kisley M.A., Noecker L., Guinther 2006, Rosenthal, Ahn & Gieger, 2011). SPD is conceptually complicated by the fact that it may include more than one phenotype and thus may not be a unitary disorder. For example, symptoms of SOR and Sensory Under-responsivity are not at all the same, and yet both fall conceptually under the framework of SPD. Regardless of its omission from the DSM-5, the body of research informs Misophonia research and should not be dismissed by those investigating this condition.

Issues in the Misophonia Literature to consider for future Research

Nature versus nurture

When conceptualizing Misophonia it is important to note that the distinction nature versus nurture (which is inexorably entwined with the "conditioned versus constitutional" paradigm) is a dated model in genetics. The interaction of genes and the environment is known to be more amorphous and less distinguishable than previously thought. Gene regulation (in which genes can be turned on or off according to environmental factors) has shifted focus off this debate and onto ways of optimizing brain plasticity in various modalities of therapeutic treatment. A pattern of disregard of this shift has already filtered through the small body of Misophonia literature, and it is important to pursue further research within this current gene regulation (or nature via nurture paradigm).

People/Body Noises versus Repetitive Noises

This is another confusing issue. The Jastreboff's conceptualized Misophonia as a condition in which individuals react aversively to "pattern-based" noises that were often but not always related to particular people. Misophonia sufferers report numerous "triggers" that are not necessarily person/body-oriented, such as "pencil tapping," "basket-ball bouncing," "keyboard typing," "environmental stimuli," "birds singing," "pen clicking," etc. (e.g. Wu, Lewin, Murphy, & Storch, 2014; Edelstein, Brang, Rouw, & Ramachandran, 2013; Schröder, Vulink, and Denys, 2013). This is highly misleading at the same time, as it may demonstrate the sufferers' difficulty differentiating the sound and the person(s) associated with the sounds. This confusion may also reflect the perpetual challenge in research related to parsing out the interactive physiological, cognitive, emotional, and processes that combine with relational dynamics to explain human behavior.

Future Research

As is always the case, cross-disciplinary research promises the most efficient and utile way to explore the underlying physiologic processes that interact with cognitive and emotional phenomena, ultimately manifesting as observable behavior. This is especially true of Misophonia, which is a newly named disorder. Yet, numerous individuals with the symptoms of Misophonia have clearly been suffering for much longer than awareness of the named disorder suggests. Consequently, it makes sense to integrate cross-disciplinary bodies of research that have addressed these and similar symptoms. At the same time, focusing in on the very specific symptoms of Misophonia will hopefully allow for research that translates into treatment.

Research Funding

Over the past year of my life, the topic of research has become an important one. Every day I am faced with the reality that soon enough, the well will run dry for funding. Misophonia is not in the DSM-5 and even conditions that are, find trouble getting any money. I have seen a lot of people complain about this. I've listened to their worries, and heard many simply respond that they are irate. But, as Jennifer so often points out - if we want this disorder researched it is quite simply "up to us".

What? That's ghastly. How can we, the people, and sufferers, be held accountable for a solution? It's actually simple: researchers can only go where the money is. There's overhead, bills to be paid, and the world has to run on somebody's dime. This does not mean that there are no researchers that care. This doesn't even mean that the governments or health organizations wouldn't help if they could. That isn't the point. Currently resources are being pointed at conditions that have known fatal causes and implications. Misophonia is new to many, and unheard of to most.

In the modern era we are simply blessed with technology and resources at our hand. It is simpler to access information. We are able to connect with sufferers across the world and share our stories. So, we can also share our worries, and we can band together in order to research this disorder and even find a cure. It won't come over night, but it's not going to come at all if we don't try.

On Dr. Brout's website, www.misophonia-research.com, you'll find information about researchers that are currently investigating Misophonia. Yes, they exist, but they need to be supported if we want them to continue.

Sometimes people that feel trapped will spend most of their time complaining about what should happen. However, the truth is: it never will until you help it along. Misophonia Research isn't going to just pop up. It takes skilled, meaningful, and perpetual efforts of people like Dr. Brout. If Jennifer doesn't have people that are willing to help fund these researchers - there will be no research. After all, the world works on a system dependent on funds. Whether they like it or not, they must go where the money goes.

The following is a message from Dr. Brout:

The National Institute of Health (NIH) and its sub-division, the National Institute of Mental Health, NIMH) is our largest granting organization for funding research for disorders such as misophonia. However, the NIMH lacks financial resources, and misophonia is not even on the "radar". So, we have to turn misfortune into opportunity.

How? For the first time we can choose our own researchers and we can have relationships with them! In the past researchers have been bound by the decisions of these government agencies and unless private funding was available, were mostly only able to study disorders that were in the accepted diagnostic manuals (currently, the DSM-5 and ICD-10). Not anymore.

Yes, those were our tax dollars at work, but how much say did you have in what was being researched, or how it was being researched?

United We Stand

I have always had a unique place right at the junction of this system, as a sufferer, parent, psychologist, fund-raiser, and donor. However, we need for all of us to do what we can, no matter how small or how large.

Together we can support this network of excellent researchers, and add to the network. We can also make sure that the researchers we work with are studying what is important to us, the sufferers.

IMNR does not accept donations. We are Misophonia sufferers and families of sufferers who help researchers we believe in raise money for research that we believe in. We only work with researchers we trust, who take us seriously and who care about us as individuals.

Dr. Jennifer Jo-Brout

Jennifer has pulled together some amazing researchers,

including top Neuroscientist Joe Ledoux. These are not your basement researchers - they are the people that will help us to put together the often jagged pieces of the larger sensory puzzle. Research is not free and it is not cheap. But, there are enough people now that are suffering that can pool together and help raise awareness and of course, help to donate to the cause.

At Misophonia International and Misophonia Research we will always be coming up with new and innovative ways to promote the research community. But, we can't do this alone. In order to succeed we need people that are willing to get on board.

As said by Napoleon Hill, "The starting point of all achievement is desire". In order to have steady Misophonia research as a community we must first desire that the research be done. The time for action is now, yesterday, and tomorrow.

Accommodations

If you have Misophonia, there may be accomodations available to you. Since Misophonia is a rare, or lesser-known disorder, you may need to explain it to your doctor first.

Proper accomodations will be between you and your doctor. Dr. Jennifer Jo-Brout has kindly shared a letter that she wrote to help a sufferer acquire accomodations. Then, Dr. Linda Girgis (M.D.) explains how she reacts to rare conditions.

The following is an example of an accommodations letter, written by Dr. Brout. While you may not use this letter for your own purposes, you may bring it to your physician as a guiding point.

This letter may aid you in explaining misophonia to your doctor, and in-turn, help to explain to a boss or teacher. All names have been omitted. Please realize that this was initially a letter used to receive accommodations for a student at an academic institution.

To Whom It May Concern:

I am writing to you on behalf of [Name Omitted]. [Name Omitted] suffers from a newly termed disorder, Misophonia. Misophonia is related to a better-known condition, Sensory Processing Disorder and is rapidly gaining recognition by audiologists, psychologists and within the allied health and mental health fields.

Unfortunately, we are only commencing the study of the overlap between these two disorders, neither, of which have a code in the Diagnostic and Statistical Manual (DSMV) or the International Classification of Diseases (ICD-10). Unfortunately, the processes of placing a newly described disorder in these diagnostic manuals is a lengthy process (often taking up to ten years while waiting for revisions).

Sadly, this leaves sufferers without diagnostic codes, and with the inability to validate their condition to others. It is a terrible "loophole" in the medical and mental health system, in which [Name Omitted] and many others presently have to deal with regarding healthcare and disability accommodations.

Therefore, as both an advocate and doctor at the forefront of this research dedicated to these related disorders I am writing to you in an effort to briefly explain [Name Omitted]'s problems and suggest accommodations that you will hopefully be willing to put into place for her. I am a School Psychologist and do understand the difficulty in making individual accommodations, especially at the University level. However, on behalf of the International Misophonia Research Network, I thank you for any assistance you will provide. Below is an explanation of the disorder, followed by suggested accommodations.

Explanation of Disorder

The term Misophonia literally means "hatred of sound.

Rather, they have highly aversive reactions to specific pat-terned-based sounds, and some are also over-responsive to visual stimuli.

Individuals with these kinds of auditory and visual over-responsivity (similar to what has been known as Sensory Pro-cessing Disorder, subtype, SOR) have demonstrated autonomic arousal and decreased habituation in neuroscience and physi-ologic studies since 1999. What does this mean for [Name Omitted]?

When [Name Omitted] encounters everyday auditory (and visual stimuli) that most people would not notice, her brain misperceives, or processes this stimuli as though it were dan-gerous. As a result, she experiences physiological arousal up to and including what we all know of as the flight/flight reaction. This is not something that is within [Name Omitted]'s control, and is part of an involuntary autonomic nervous system re-sponse. This happens in milliseconds without conscious media-tion.

As such, sufferers, feel bombarded by both noise and vi-sual stimuli. Once this bombardment occurs [Name Omitted] may feel a variety of physical discomforts such as nausea, diz-ziness, as well as what one might describe as increasing mental and physical tension and a more subjective need to "flee" (or more simply stated) leave the place in which offending stimuli exists. Again, this is a fight/flight reaction that is beyond [Name Omitted]' control. If she is unable to "flee" or leave the environment in order to get away from the aversive stimuli, her adrenaline level continues to elevate, and other hormonal and physiological changes related to the fight/flight response occur, culminating in what many people describe as experience, "a severe anxiety attack", "rage", or "panic".

In addition, 15 years of research on individuals with Sensory Over-Responsivity has also shown a deficit in habituation. That is, once the fight/flight system is set off, the part of the nervous system that is normally activated in order to put the "brakes" on fight/flight does not act efficiently. Thus, for [Name Omitted], normal everyday sensory stimuli is overloading and causes her to become severely dysregulated, but also the way her particular nervous system works disables her ability to calm down.

Unfortunately, it is impossible to predict what auditory or other sensory stimuli might cause reactivity. Often the stimuli vary, and change over time. In addition, levels of reactivity may vary from day to day and in association with stress, rest and other daily living factors. To date, there is no cure for this condition. Occupational Therapy has helped in regard to some elements of Sensory Processing Disorder. However, there is as of yet no treatment for auditory of visual over-responsivity, or most certainly not for the condition now described as Misophonia.

As such, it is extraordinarily difficult for people with this condition to lead functional lives. The problem is not simply one of dealing with the continually overloaded and dysregulated system. The problem extends to the toll this takes on one's body. Individuals with this problem often become extremely tired, or conversely develop sleep difficulty. They may also suffer from depression because this is a difficult condition with which to live, with no treatment and little understanding within even the medical community as of yet.

There are times that exposing oneself to an environment full of sensory stimuli is both physically and psychologically overwhelming to the extent that recent research describes many sufferers living very isolated lives, and others often feeling the need to stay at home where they can control the sounds and light levels (for example).

Both SPD/SOR research and the new Misophonia research both suggest that severity of the disorder runs on a continuum, with some people experiencing it as much more severe than others and with possible variations throughout the lifespan.

At this point in time there are no validated severity measures from which a doctor can determine an individuals' level of life impairment or functioning, and most sufferers (as well as psychologists) are using practical daily living skills and management plans to try to assist until further research on the etiology and treatment of this disorder is developed.

Recommendations

[Name Omitted] should to take quizzes and tests in a

room separate from others. This will allow her to minimize sensory stimuli to which she may react.

[Name Omitted] should be allowed to leave the classroom for small breaks when needed. Sensory stimuli is cumulative and therefore frequent breaks can be helpful

However, she should also be given the following options whenever
possible:

[Name Omitted] should also be allowed to digitally record her classes. This would ensure that she would benefit from all class lecture if she is unable to attend class, needs to leave class frequently and/or misses educational opportunity during class due to the distraction often caused by her condition

Considering the sensory and misophonia issues coupled with her history of anxiety and depression (and the ways in which these disorders interact and overlap) [Name Omitted] is going to need advocacy from within the school in regard to explaining her condition to her professors. Given the physical and mentally impairing effects of this condition and related anxiety and depression, considerations should be given to [Name Omitted] if she is unable to attend class.

Following are suggestions for this:

In the event that [Name Omitted] misses class her note-taker should give her class note and ideally that same person would be responsible for also recording the class so that [Name Omitted] can keep up with class discussions

Dr. Jennifer Jo-Brout, IMRN

The following interview is with Dr. Linda. She is an MD in the Unites States and has a special interest in rare disorders.

A Doctor's Opinion on Rare Diseases

Dr. Linda Girgis and I met over Twitter. Her interest in rare disorders led to conversations about Misophonia. Dr. Linda hadn't heard about Misophonia until our discourse, but her interest in rare diseases caught my eye. After-all, we need doctors like Linda. In this interview we talk about SERMO, and Dr. Linda shares her compassionate approach to rare diseases and treatment.

Could you tell us about your affiliation with SERMO? Who are they/what do they do?

SERMO is the largest online network exclusive to only physicians. On the site, we collaborate about cases and talk about general things in healthcare. And some socializing as well. If I have a difficult case I need help with, I can create a post on SERMO and get online help from my colleagues.

I am a medical advisor for SERMO, they want to be sure they keep physicians' voices in what they do. I also am one of their "hub ambassadors": I write articles for the obesity and rare disease hubs. These are learning hubs for educational purposes. And I am one of their blog columnists.

You write about rare diseases and medical conditions:

What are some of the rarest you've come across in your practice?

I have had a few rare disease patients in my practice. The rarest was Moyamoya syndrome*.

As a doctor, when a patient comes to you with a rare disorder that you have never heard of it, how might you handle it?

Most of the rare disease patients I have seen are already seeing specialists and I am treating them for other problems (acute infection, etc). I will research the disease and try to educate myself about their disease. And, I will try to ensure that they are indeed seeing the right specialists for their disease.

Since they are harder to diagnose, do you find it a challenge to get patients to open up about their rare disorders? Have you ever felt a patient was holding back in fear of being judged?

Yes, this is a big problem. Many rare disease patients that I have treated feel that people don't understand them. And the truth is, science doesn't because many of these diseases we just don't know enough about. I feel some xof rare disease patients do feel stigmatized, judged, and misunderstood. I find that parents of kids with rare diseases are more likely to open up about their child's rare disease.

What advice can you give to patients that are scared to confront their doctor with a condition that you, or many others, have never heard of?

It is very important that your doctor know everything about your medical condition. If we don't, we will not be able to give you the best care. As doctors, we are trained to be non-judgmental. However, doctors are human and this may not always be true. If you are seeing a doctor who you feel you cannot be completely open with, you need to find a new one. You need to trust your doctor and vice versa.

If I have a patient with a condition that I never heard of, I will tell them so. And ask them to tell me how it has affected them. I will then do my best to try to learn as much as I can about that disease. If I am to give my patients my best medical advice, I need to know as much as possible.

And, when I don't know what to do, I will try to find the best available specialist to help.

Do you believe the current system in the US properly cares for patients with rare and unheard of conditions?

No. We are not even doing a good job giving proper care to patients with common chronic conditions. All too often, insurance companies are denying diagnostic tests and medications. And this is especially worse for rare disease patients who may require unusual diagnostic tests to diagnose their conditions.

Also, research monies are going to the most lucrative disease and little is being spent towards researching rare disease.

If a patient came to you with Misophonia, a condition that is nearly impossible to diagnose, how would you help a patient to acquire accommodations from either work or school?
I write many letters of medical necessity for my patients for various conditions, including work and school accommodations. I would ask the pt what would help them to be able to function better and feel more comfortable at work or school. And then I would send a letter outlining what accommodations are necessary.

Do you believe there is a large stigma that still affects persons that have rare disorders?
I believe there is. And I think until; more research is done and we start understanding these disease better, it will unfortunately remain.

Is there anything else you might like to add?
I am very passionate about rare disease patients. I have written articles about how I believe they are being harmed in our current health system. Our healthcare system (3rd party payers, governmental plans) are more geared to cost savings and not giving patients the best care. And rare disease patients are being hurt because of this.

It is scary enough having a disease. But, when it is a disease that few other people have and even doctors don't understand it, it is horrifying.

I think we should all try to put ourselves in the shoes of a rare disease pt for a few moments and imagine how scary it must be .And then, we all need to step up and do better by them, from doctors to researchers to teachers to society. All of us, individually and professionally.

* Moyamoya disease is a rare, progressive cerebrovascular disorder caused by blocked arteries at the base of the brain in an area called the basal ganglia.

Rights And Legal Information

This chapter will focus on any rights and legal implications that a person with Misophonia should be aware of. I will do my best to give you information on accessibility rights, and the implications of certain bodies denying you of your rights. It is important to note that my home country is Canada, so any information from other countries is purely based on research, not first-hand experience. This chapter merely serves as an outline of important considerations. Please see your local laws and medical practices regarding conditions such as Misophonia. Most countries have something in place for accessibility. This chapter will also feature links to resources. Part of the problem comes with whether or not Misophonia is classified as a disability. Through awareness, we will hopefully help medical communities and governments understand that Misophonia is a life-altering condition that should be classified as a disability.

If you are looking for accessibility services at your school or workplace, you should first communicate with your employer or guidance counselor and see what they have in place. Some employers may have better accommodations than others. At the very least, you should inform them that you might need special accommodations. If your employer does not have a system in place, or requires more documentation, please see your local laws in regards to accessibility. There is a large chance that you will need to contact a doctor to get a form of documentation. This is not meant to be a full guide, but merely a starting place.

Excerpts of legal acts can be found near the end of the book, in the appendixes.

United States

The United States has an act that aims to protect all persons with

disabilities. In the Gale Encyclopedia of American law, this is explained.

The Americans with Disabilities Act (ADA), which was enacted in 1990, is a landmark civil rights law. It has been called the "Bill of Rights" for persons with disabilities, who make up approximately 20 percent of the U.S. population. Prior to its enactment, a patchwork of federal, state, and local laws attempted to eliminate disability discrimination. That approach proved ineffective. The act prohibits discrimination against persons with disabilities in employment, public accommodations, transportation, and telecommunications (Batten 396)

Canada

Canada has the Charter of Rights and Freedoms, in this charter it is proclaimed that no citizen will be discriminated against based on a disability.

15. (1) Every individual is equal before and under the law and has the right to the equal protection and equal benefit of the law without discrimination and, in particular, without discrimination based on race, national or ethnic origin, colour, religion, sex, age or mental or physical disability (The Constitu-

tion Act, 1983 www.laws-lois.justice.gc.ca)

Since there are several provinces/territories in Canada, and a lot of different practices for each, these are the resources for each. Many of the policies are similar, but you should use the resource for your home province or territory, in case of discrepancies. Every province must ensure that their employers are meeting the basic standards for human rights, and that they are obeying the charter. This does not mean that they will

have the same practices and standards.

British Columbia

www.bcands.bc.ca/wp-content/uploads/Accessibility-2014-BC-

Government-Release.pdf

Alberta

www.albertahumanrights.ab.ca

Saskatchewan

www.canlii.org/en/sk/laws/stat/ss-1979-c-s-24.1/latest

Manitoba

www.gov.mb.ca/dio/discussionpaper/discussion_w5

www.canlii.org/en/mb/laws/stat/ccsm-c-h175/latest/

Ontario

http://www.canlii.org/en/on/laws/stat/so-2005-c-11/latest/

Quebec

http://www.canlii.org/en/qc/laws/stat/rsq-c-e-20.1/latest/

New Brunswick

http://www.canlii.org/en/nb/laws/stat/rsnb-1973-c-h-11/
latest/

Nova Scotia

http://www.canlii.org/en/ns/laws/stat/rsns-1989-c-214/
latest/

Prince Edward Island

http://www.canlii.org/en/pe/laws/stat/rspei-1988-c-h-12/
latest/

Newfoundland and Labrador

http://www.canlii.org/en/nl/laws/stat/snl-2010-c-h-13.1/
latest/

Northwest Territories

http://www.canlii.org/en/nt/laws/stat/snwt-2002-c-18/
latest/

Yukon Territory

http://www.canlii.org/en/yk/laws/stat/rsy-2002-c-116/
latest/

Nunavut

http://www.canlii.org/en/nu/laws/stat/snu-2003-c-12/
latest/

Australia

Australia operates under the Disability Discrimination Act

1992. This means that the entire country must consider the implications of this act. The following is an excerpt from the act:

(1) It is unlawful for an employer or a person acting or purporting to act on behalf of an employer to discriminate against a person on the ground of the other person's disability: (a) in the arrangements made for the purpose of determining who should be offered employment; or (b) in determining who should be offered employment; or (c) in the terms or conditions on which employment is offered.

(2) It is unlawful for an employer or a person acting or purporting to act (Disability Discrimination Act 1992).

Australian laws can be found at the following links www.comlaw.gov.au

UK

The UK has the Equality Act 2010 that outlines laws regarding discrimination and disabilities. According to the document, "(1) A person (P) has a disability if—

(a) P has a physical or mental impairment, and (b) the impairment has a substantial and long-term adverse effect on P's ability to carry out normal day-to-day activities" (Equality Act 2010).

These laws can be found at www.legislation.gov.uk

Appendices

Appendix 1: The American Disabilities Act 1990

In text-citation: (The American Disabilities Act 1990, acquired from Batten 397-433)

Note: This is not the entire document, merely sections that have been deemed relevant.

TITLE I–EMPLOYMENT

SEC. 102. DISCRIMINATION.

(a) GENERAL RULE.—No covered entity shall discriminate against a qualified individual with a disability because of the disability of such individual in regard to job application procedures, the hiring, advancement, or discharge of employees, employee compensation,

job training, and other terms, conditions, and privileges of employment. (b) CONSTRUCTION.—As used in subsection (a), the term "discriminate" includes—

(1) limiting, segregating, or classifying a job applicant or employee in a way that adversely affects the opportunities or status of such applicant or employee because of the disability of such applicant or employee;

(2) participating in a contractual or other arrangement or relationship that has the effect of subjecting a covered entity's qualified applicant or employee with a disability to the discrimination prohibited by this title (such relationship includes

a relationship with an employment or referral agency, labor union, an organization providing fringe benefits to an employee of the covered entity, or an organization providing training and apprenticeship programs);

(3) utilizing standards, criteria, or methods of administration—

(A) that have the effect of discrimination on the basis of disability; or (B) that perpetuate the discrimination of others who are subject to common administrative control;

(4) excluding or otherwise denying equal jobs or benefits to a qualified individual because of the known disability of an individual with whom the qualified individual is known to have a relationship or association;

(5) (A) not making reasonable accommodations to the known physical or mental limitations of an otherwise qualified individual with a disability who is an applicant or employee, unless such covered entity can demonstrate that the accommodation would impose an undue hardship on the operation of the business of such covered entity; or

(B) denying employment opportunities to a job applicant or employee who is an otherwise qualified individual with a disability, if such denial is based on the need of such covered entity to make reasonable accommodation to the physical or mental impairments of the employee or applicant;

(6) using qualification standards, employment tests or

other selection criteria that screen out or tend to screen out an individual with a disability or a class of individuals with disabilities unless the standard, test or other selection criteria, as used by the covered entity, is shown to be job-related for the position in question and is consistent with business necessity; and (7) failing to select and administer tests concerning employment in the most effective manner to ensure that, when such test is administered to a job applicant or employee who has a disability that impairs sensory, manual, or speaking skills, such test results accurately reflect the skills, aptitude, or whatever other factor of such applicant or employee that such test purports to measure, rather than reflecting the impaired sensory, manual, or speaking skills of such employee or applicant (except where such skills are the factors that the test purports to measure).

(c) MEDICAL EXAMINATIONS AND INQUIRIES.—

(1) IN GENERAL.—The prohibition against discrimination as referred to in subsection (a) shall include medical examinations and inquiries.

(2) PREEMPLOYMENT.—

(A) PROHIBITED EXAMINATION OR INQUIRY.—Except as provided in paragraph (3), a covered entity shall not conduct a medical examination or make inquiries of a job applicant as to whether such applicant is an individual with a disability or as to the nature or severity of such disability. (B) ACCEPTABLE INQUIRY.—A covered entity may make pre-employment inquiries into the ability of an applicant to perform job related functions. (3) EMPLOYMENT ENTRANCE EXAMINATION.—A covered entity may require a medical examination after an offer of employment has been made to a job applicant and prior to the commencement of the

employment duties of such applicant, and may condition an offer of employment on the results of such examination, if—

(A) all entering employees are subjected to such an examination regardless of disability;

(B) information obtained regarding the medical condition or history of the applicant is collected and maintained on separate forms and in separate medical files and is treated as a confidential medical record, except that —

(i) supervisors and managers may be informed regarding necessary restrictions on the work or duties of the employee and necessary accommodations;

(ii) first aid and safety personnel may be informed, when appropriate, if the disability might require emergency treatment; and

(iii) government officials investigating compliance with this Act shall be provided relevant information on request; and

(C) the results of such examination are used only in accordance with this title.

(4) EXAMINATION AND INQUIRY.—

(A) PROHIBITED EXAMINATIONS AND INQUIRIES.—A covered entity shall not require a medical examination and shall not make inquiries of an employee as to whether such employee is an individual with a disability or as to the nature or severity of the disability, unless such examination or inquiry is shown to be job related and consistent with business necessity.

(B) ACCEPTABLE EXAMINATIONS AND INQUIRIES.—A covered entity may conduct voluntary medical examinations, including voluntary medical histories, which are part of an employee health program available to employees at that work site. A covered entity may make inquiries into the ability of an employee to perform job-related functions.

(C) REQUIREMENT.—Information obtained under subparagraph (B) regarding the medical condition or history of any employee are subject to the requirements of subparagraphs (B) and (C) of paragraph (3).

SEC. 103. DEFENSES.

(a) IN GENERAL.—It may be a defense to a charge of discrimination under this Act that an alleged application of qualification standards, tests, or selection criteria that screen out or tend to screen out or otherwise deny a job or benefit to an individual with a disability has been shown to be job-

related and consistent with business necessity, and such performance cannot be accomplished by reasonable accommodation, as required under this title.

(b) QUALIFICATION STANDARDS.—The term "qualification standards" may include a requirement that an individual shall not pose a direct threat to the health or safety of other individuals in the workplace.

(c) RELIGIOUS ENTITIES.—

(1) IN GENERAL.—This title shall not prohibit a religious corporation, association, educational institution, or society from giving preference in employment to individuals of a particular religion to perform work connected with the carrying on by such corporation, association, educational institution, or society of its activities.

(2) RELIGIOUS TENETS REQUIREMENT.—Under this title, a religious organization may require that all applicants and employees conform to the religious tenets of such organization.

(d) LIST OF INFECTIOUS AND COMMUNICABLE DIS-EASES.—

(1) IN GENERAL.—The Secretary of Health and Human Services, not later than 6 months after the date of enactment of this Act, shall—

(A) review all infectious and communicable diseases which may be transmitted through handling the food supply;

(B) publish a list of infectious and communicable diseases which are transmitted through handling the food supply;

(C) publish the methods by which such diseases are transmitted; and

(D) widely disseminate such information regarding the list of diseases and their modes of transmissibility to the general public.

Such list shall be updated annually.

(2) APPLICATIONS.—In any case in which an individual has an infectious or communicable disease that is transmitted to others through the handling of food, that is included on the list developed by the Secretary of Health and Human Services under paragraph (1), and which cannot be eliminated by reasonable accommodation, a covered entity may refuse to assign or continue to assign such individual to a job involving food handling.

(3) CONSTRUCTION.—Nothing in this Act shall be construed to preempt, modify, or amend any State, county, or local law, ordinance, or regulation applicable to food handling which is designed to protect the public

health from individuals who pose a significant risk to the health or safety of others, which cannot be eliminated by reasonable accommodation, pursuant to the list of infectious or communicable diseases and the modes of transmissibility published by the Secretary of Health and Human Services.

Appendix 2 CANADIAN CONSTITUTION ACT, 1982

Citation: (Canadian Charter of Rights and Freedoms)

Note: This is not the entire document, merely sections that have been deemed relevant

PART I

CANADIAN CHARTER OF RIGHTS AND FREEDOMS

Whereas Canada is founded upon principles that recognize

the supremacy of God and the rule of law:

GUARANTEE OF RIGHTS AND FREEDOMS

Marginal note: Rights and freedoms in Canada

1. The Canadian Charter of Rights and Freedoms guarantees the rights and freedoms set out in it subject only to such reasonable limits prescribed by law as can be demonstrably justified in a free and democratic society.

FUNDAMENTAL FREEDOMS

Marginal note: Fundamental freedoms

2. Everyone has the following fundamental freedoms:

- (a) freedom of conscience and religion;
- (b) freedom of thought, belief, opinion and expression,

including

freedom of the press and other media of communication;

- (c) freedom of peaceful assembly; and
- (d) freedom of association.

LEGAL RIGHTS

Marginal note: Life, liberty and security of person

7. Everyone has the right to life, liberty and security of the person and the right not to be deprived thereof except in accordance with the principles of fundamental justice.

Marginal note: Search or seizure

12. Everyone has the right not to be subjected to any cruel and unusual treatment or punishment.

EQUALITY RIGHTS

Marginal note: Equality before and under law and equal protection and benefit of law

- 15. (1) Every individual is equal before and under the law and has the right to the equal protection and equal benefit of the law without discrimination and, in particular, without discrimination based on race, national or ethnic origin, colour, religion, sex, age or mental or physical disability.

- Marginal note: Affirmative action programs

(2) Subsection (1) does not preclude any law, program or activity that has as its object the amelioration of conditions of disadvantaged individuals or groups including those that are disadvantaged because of race, national or ethnic origin, colour, religion, sex, age or mental or physical disability.

ENFORCEMENT

Marginal note: Enforcement of guaranteed rights and freedoms

- 24. (1) Anyone whose rights or freedoms, as guaranteed by this Charter, have been infringed or denied may apply to a court of competent jurisdiction to obtain such remedy as the court considers appropriate and just in the circumstances.

- Marginal note: Exclusion of evidence bringing administration of justice into disrepute

(2) Where, in proceedings under subsection (1), a court concludes that evidence was obtained in a manner that infringed or denied any rights or freedoms guaranteed by this Charter, the evidence shall be excluded if it is established that,

having regard to all the circumstances, the admission of it in the proceedings would bring the administration of justice into disrepute.

Appendix 3 – Australian Disability Discrimination Act 1992

Citation: (Disability Discrimination Act 1992)

Note: This is not the entire document, merely sections that have been deemed relevant

Part 2—Prohibition of disability discrimination Division 1—Discrimination in work

15 Discrimination in employment

(1) It is unlawful for an employer or a person acting or purporting to act on behalf of an employer to discriminate against a person on the ground of the other person's disability:

(a) in the arrangements made for the purpose of determining who should be offered employment; or

(b) in determining who should be offered employment; or

(c) in the terms or conditions on which employment is

offered.

(2) It is unlawful for an employer or a person acting or purporting

to act on behalf of an employer to discriminate against an employee on the ground of the employee's disability:

(a) in the terms or conditions of employment that the employer affords the employee; or

(b) by denying the employee access, or limiting the employee's access, to opportunities for promotion, transfer or training, or to any other benefits associated with employment; or

(c) by dismissing the employee; or

(d) by subjecting the employee to any other detriment. (3) Neither paragraph (1)(a) nor (b) renders it unlawful for a person to discriminate against another person, on the ground of the other person's disability, in connection with employment to perform domestic duties on the premises on which the firstmentioned person resides.

16 Discrimination against commission agents

(1) It is unlawful for a principal to discriminate against a person on the ground of the person's disability:

(a) in the arrangements the principal makes for the purpose of determining who should be engaged as a commission agent; or

(b) in determining who should be engaged as a commission agent; or

(c) in the terms or conditions on which the person is engaged as a commission agent.

(2) It is unlawful for a principal to discriminate against a commission agent on the ground of the commission agent's disability:

(a) in the terms or conditions that the principal affords the commission agent as a commission agent; or

(b) by denying the commission agent access, or limiting the commission agent's access, to opportunities for promotion, transfer or training, or to any other benefits associated with the position as a commission agent; or

(c) by terminating the engagement; or

(d) by subjecting the commission agent to any other detriment.

17 Discrimination against contract workers

It is unlawful for a principal to discriminate against a contract worker on the ground of the contract worker's disability:

(a) in the terms or conditions on which the principal allows the contract worker to work; or

(b) by not allowing the contract worker to work or continue to work; or

(c) by denying the contract worker access, or limiting the contract worker's access, to any benefit associated with the work in respect of which the contract with the employer is made; or

(d) by subjecting the contract worker to any other detriment.

20 Registered organisations under the Fair Work (Registered Organisations) Act 2009

(1) It is unlawful for a registered organisation, the committee of management of a registered organisation or a member of the committee of management of a registered organisation

to discriminate against a person, on the ground of the person's disability:

(a) by refusing or failing to accept the person's application for membership; or

(b) in the terms or conditions on which the organisation is prepared to admit the person to membership.

(2) It is unlawful for a registered organisation, the committee of management of a registered organisation or a member of the committee of management of a registered organisation to discriminate against a person who is a member of the registered organisation, on the ground of the member's disability:

(a) by denying the member access or limiting the member's access, to any benefit provided by the organisation; or

(b) by depriving the member of membership or varying the terms of membership; or

(c) by subjecting the member to any other detriment.

21 Employment agencies

(1) It is unlawful for an employment agency to discriminate against a person on the ground of the person's disability:

(a) by refusing to provide the person with any of its services; or

(b) in the terms or conditions on which it offers to provide the person with any of its services; or

(c) in the manner in which it provides the person with any of its services.

(2) This Part does not require an employment agency to ensure that an employer complies with this Act.

(3) Subsection (2) does not affect the operation of section 122 (which applies if an employment agency causes, instructs, induces, aids or permits an employer to do an unlawful act).

Division 2—Discrimination in other areas 22 Education

(1) It is unlawful for an educational authority to discriminate against a person on the ground of the person's disability:

(a) by refusing or failing to accept the person's application for admission as a student; or

(b) in the terms or conditions on which it is prepared to admit the person as a student.

(2) It is unlawful for an educational authority to discriminate against a student on the ground of the student's disability:

(a) by denying the student access, or limiting the student's access, to any benefit provided by the educational authority; or

(b) by expelling the student; or

(c) by subjecting the student to any other detriment.

(2A) It is unlawful for an education provider to discriminate against

a person on the ground of the person's disability:

(a) by developing curricula or training courses having a

content that will either exclude the person from participation, or subject the person to any other detriment; or

(b) by accrediting curricula or training courses having such a content.

(3) This section does not render it unlawful to discriminate against a person on the ground of the person's disability in respect of admission to an educational institution established wholly or primarily for students who have a particular disability where the person does

Appendix 4 – UK Equality Act 2010

BE IT ENACTED by the Queen's most Excellent Majesty, by and with the advice and consent of the Lords Spiritual and Temporal, and Commons, in this present Parliament assembled, and by the authority of the same, as follows:—

6. Disability

(1) A person (P) has a disability if—

(a) P has a physical or mental impairment, and

(b) the impairment has a substantial and long-term adverse effect on P's ability to carry out normal day-to-day activities.

(2) A reference to a disabled person is a reference to a person who has a disability.

(3) In relation to the protected characteristic of disability—

(a) a reference to a person who has a particular protected characteristic is a reference to a person who has a particular disability;

(b) a reference to persons who share a protected characteristic is a reference to persons who have the same disability.

(4) This Act (except Part 12 and section 190) applies in

relation to a person who has had a disability as it applies in relation to a person who has the disability; accordingly (except in that Part and that section)—

(a) a reference (however expressed) to a person who has a disability includes a reference to a person who has had the disability, and

(b) a reference (however expressed) to a person who does not have a disability includes a reference to a person who has not had the disability. (5) A Minister of the Crown may issue guidance about matters to be taken into account in deciding any question for the purposes of subsection (1). (6) Schedule 1 (disability: supplementary provision) has effect.

Discrimination

Direct discrimination

(1) A person (A) discriminates against another (B) if, because of a protected characteristic, A treats B less favourably than A treats or would treat others.

(2) If the protected characteristic is age, A does not discriminate against B if A can show A's treatment of B to be a proportionate means of achieving a legitimate aim.

(3) If the protected characteristic is disability, and B is not a disabled person, A does not discriminate against B only because A treats or would treat disabled persons more favourably than A treats B.

(4) If the protected characteristic is marriage and civil

partnership, this section applies to a contravention of Part 5 (work) only if the treatment is because it is B who is married or a civil partner.

(5)If the protected characteristic is race, less favourable treatment includes segregating B from others.

(6)If the protected characteristic is sex—

(a)less favourable treatment of a woman includes less favourable treatment of her because she is breast-feeding;

(b)in a case where B is a man, no account is to be taken of special treatment afforded to a woman in connection with pregnancy or childbirth.

(7)Subsection (6)(a) does not apply for the purposes of Part 5 (work). (8)This section is subject to sections 17(6) and 18(7).

PROSPECTIVE

Combined discrimination: dual characteristics

(1)A person (A) discriminates against another (B) if, because of a combination of two relevant protected characteristics, A treats B less favourably than A treats or would treat a person who does not share either of those characteristics.

(2)The relevant protected characteristics are—

(a)age;

(b)disability;

(c)gender reassignment;

(d)race

(e)religion or belief;

(f) sex;

(g) sexual orientation.

(3) For the purposes of establishing a contravention of this Act by virtue of subsection (1), B need not show that A's treatment of B is direct discrimination because of each of the characteristics in the combination (taken separately).

(4) But B cannot establish a contravention of this Act by virtue of subsection (1) if, in reliance on another provision of this Act or any other enactment, A shows that A's treatment of B is not direct discrimination because of either or both of the characteristics in the combination. (5) Subsection (1) does not apply to a combination of characteristics that includes disability in circumstances where, if a claim of direct discrimination because of disability were to be brought, it would come within section 116 (special educational needs).

(6) A Minister of the Crown may by order amend this section so as to— (a) make further provision about circumstances in which B can, or in which B cannot, establish a contravention of this Act by virtue of subsection (1); (b) specify other circumstances in which subsection (1) does not apply. (7) The references to direct discrimination are to a contravention of this Act by virtue of section 13.

15 Discrimination arising from disability

(1) A person (A) discriminates against a disabled person (B) if—

(a) A treats B unfavourably because of something arising in consequence of B's disability, and

(b) A cannot show that the treatment is a proportionate means of achieving a legitimate aim.

(2) Subsection (1) does not apply if A shows that A did not know, and could not reasonably have been expected to know, that B had the disability.

Bibliography

(Australian) "Disability Discrimination Act 1992"

Batten, Donna. "The American Disabilities Act 1990", Gale Encyclopedia of American Law. 2011. Gale Group. 397-433. eBook.

Bernstein, R. E., Angell, K. L., & Dehle, C. M. "A brief course of cognitive behavioural therapy for the treatment of misophonia: A case example". The Cognitive Behaviour Therapist, 6, 1-13.

"Canadian Charter of Rights and Freedoms"

CAMH. Beyond the Label: An Educational Kit to Promote Awareness and Understanding of the Impact of Stigma on People Living with Concurrent Mental Health and Substance Use Problems. Toronto, ON, CAN: Centre for Addiction and Mental Health, 2005. ProQuest ebrary. Web. 24 May 2015.

Edelstein, Mirem, David Brand, Romke Rouw, and Vilayanur S. Ramachandran. "Misophonia: physiological investigations and case descriptions". Frontiers In Human Neuroscience,.

Johnston, J. M., & Pennypacker, H. S. Strategies and tactics of behavioral research. New York, NY: Rutledge. 2009.

Johnson, M. 50 cases of misophonia using the MMP, 2014.

Kuebler-Ross, Elisabeth. On Death and Dying. , 1969. Print.

Moss, Michael. Salt Sugar Fat: How The Food Giants Hooked Us. NY: Random House, 2013. eBook.

Yudkin, John. Pure, White and Deadly. London: Penguin Books, 1986. eBook.

(UK) "Equality Act 2010"REFERENCES

Ahn, R., Miller, L. J., Milberger, S., &McIntosh, D. N. (2004). Prevalence of parents' perceptions of sensory processing disorders among kindergarten children. American Journal of Occupational Therapy, 58 (3), 287-302.

Alvarado J.C, Vaughan J.W, Stanford T.R., and Stein B.E. (2007). Multisensory Versus Unisensory Integration: Contrasting Modes in the Superior Colliculus. Journal of Neurophysiology 97, 3193–3205.

Ben-Sasson, A., Carter, A.S., & Briggs Gowan, M.J. (2009). Sensory over- responsivity in elementary school: prevalence and social-emotional correlates. Journal of Abnormal Child Psychology, 37, 705-716.

Ben-Sasson, A., Carter, A.S., & Briggs-Gowan, M.J. (2010). The development of sensory over-responsivity from infancy to elementary school. Journal of Abnormal Child Psychology, 38 (8), 1193-1202.

Carter, A.S., Ben-Sasson, A., & Briggs-Gowan, M.J. (2011). Sensory over- responsivity, psychopathology, and family impairment in school-aged children. Journal of the American Academy of Child & Adolescent Psychiatry, 50 (12), 1210-1219.

Davies, P.L., Chang, W-P., & Gavin, W.J. (2009). Maturation of Sensory Gating Performance in Children with and without Sensory Processing Disorders. International Journal of Psychophysiology, 72,187-197.

Davies P.L., Chang, W.P., & Gavin, W.J. (2010). Middle and late latency ERP components discriminate between adults, typical children, and children with sensory processing disorders. Frontiers in Integrative Neuroscience, 4, 16.

Davies, P.L. & Gavin, W.J. (2007). Validating the diagnosis of Sensory Processing Disorders using EEG technology.

American Journal of Occupational Therapy, 61 (2), 176-189.

Edelstein M, Brang D, Rouw R, Ramachandran VS (2013). Misophonia: physiological investigations and case descriptions.. Frontiers in Human Neuroscience 2013;7(296), 1-11, doi: 10.3389/fnhum.2013.00296

Gavin, W. J., Dotseth, A., Roush, K. K., Smith, C. A., Spain, H. D., & Davies, P. L. (2011). Electroencephalography in children with and without sensory processing disorders during auditory perception. American Journal of Occupational Therapy, 65, 370–377

Goldsmith, H.H., Van Hulle, C.A., Arneson, C.L., Schreiber, J.E., & Gernsbacher, M.A. (2006). A population-based twin study of parentally reported tactile and auditory defensiveness in young children. Journal of Abnormal Child Psychology, 34 (3), 393-407.

Jastreboff MM, Jastreboff PJ. (2001) Hyperacusis. Audiology Online. www.audiologyonline.com/articles/hyperacusis-1223.

Jastreboff PJ, Jastreboff MM. (2006) Tinnitus retraining therapy: a different view on tinnitus. International Journal of Pediatric Otorhinolaryngology, 68(1):23–29.

Keuler, M.M., Schmidt, N.L., Van Hulle, C.A., Lemery-Chalfant, K., & Goldsmith, H.H. (2011). Sensory overresponsivity: prenatal risk factors and temperamental contributions. Journal of Development & Behavioral Pediatrics, 32 (7), 533-541.

Kisley M.A., Noecker L., Guinther P.M. (2004). Comparison of sensory gating to mismatch negativity and self-reported perceptual phenomena in healthy adults. International Journal of Psychophysiology, 41, 604–612. DOI: 10.1111/j.1469-8986.2004.00191.x

Lane, S.J., Reynolds, S., & Thacker, L. (2010). Sensory over-responsivity and ADHD: differentiating using elec-trodermal responses, cortisol, and anxiety. Frontiers in Integrative Neuroscience, 4 (8),1-14. doi:10.3389/fnint.2010.00008

McIntosh DN, Miller LJ, Shyu V, Hagerman. (1999). Sensory-modulation disruption, electrodermal responses, and functional behaviors. Developmental Medicine & Child Neurology. 41, 608-615.

Owen, J.P., Marco E.J., Desai S., Fourie E., Harris J., Hill S.S.,

Arnett A.B., Mukherjee P., (2103) Abnormal white matter microstructure in children with sensory processing disorders. NeuroImage: Clinical, 2, 844–853.

Rosenthal, M.Z., Ahn, R. & Geiger , P.J. (2011). Reactivity to Sensations in Borderline Personality Disorder: A Preliminary Study. Journal of Personality Disorders: Vol. 25, No. 5, pp. 715-721.

Schaaf, R.C., Miller, L.J., Seawell, D., & O'Keefe, S. (2003). Children with disturbances in sensory processing: A pilot study examining the role of the parasympathetic nervous system. American Journal of Occupational Therapy, 57.

Schneider, M.L., Moore, C.F., Larson, J.A., Barr, C.S., DeJesus, O.T., & Roberts, A.D. (2009). Timing of moderate level of prenatal alcohol exposure influences gene expression of sensory processing behavior in rhesus monkeys. Frontiers in Integrative Neuroscience, 3, 30.

Schröder A, Vulink N, Denys D. (2013) Misophonia: diagnostic criteria for a new psychiatric disorder. PLoS One, 8 (1). doi:10.1371/journal.pone. 0054706.

Tavassoli T., Miller L.J., Schoen S.A., Nielsen D.M., Baron-Cohen S. (2014). Sensory over-responsivity in adults with autism spectrum conditions. Autism, 18 (4), 28-32.

Van Hulle, C.A., Schmidt, N.L., & Goldsmith, H.H. (2012). Is sensory over- responsivity distinguishable from childhood behavior problems? A phenotypic and genetic analysis. Journal of Child Psychology and Psychiatry, 53 (1), 64-72.

Wu MS, Lewin AB, Murphy TK, Storch EA. (2014) Misophonia: incidence, phenomenology, and clinical correlates in an undergraduate student sample. Journal of Clinical Psychology. Published online April 17. doi: 10.1002/jclp.22098

About The Author

Shaylynn Hayes is a 22 year old
writer, graphic/webdesigner, and
student. For her first few years of University Shaylynn studied English Lit, Irish
Studies, and Political Science (St. Thomas,
Fredericton). However, Shaylynn has now
changed her major
to Psychology with a double-major
in Political Science. Misophonia has

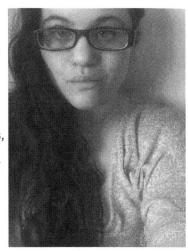

created both trials and tribulations. It is due to Misophonia that she ended
up switching schools, but it is also the reason she has been able to focus
her voice and try to help others that struggle with the disorder. A year ago
Shaylynn formed **MisophoniaAwareness.org** and continues to update the
site when new and more current information is available. However, this has
become a secondary project to an even wider, more international initiative.
Alongside Dr. Jennifer Brout, Shaylynn runs the News site and Magazine,
Misophonia International. The site focuses on Research, Coping, and Awareness for the disorder. Shaylynn has also been actively involved in the web
management and development of Dr. Brout's research page, **Misophonia-
Research.com** .

What used to be a life-ruining disorder has become an interesting and defin-
ing adventure that has proven that the things that are "ruining our life" may
very well be creating a new, interesting life in the place of the old.

17812689R00121

Printed in Poland
by Amazon Fulfillment
Poland Sp. z o.o., Wrocław